Contents

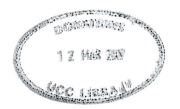
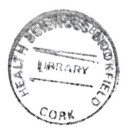

51715479C

Glossary

ADON	Assistant Director of Nursing
Atypical Antipsychotic Drugs	Antipsychotic drugs which are newer and more expensive than standard antipsychotics and produce different side effects. In particular, they give fewer neuromuscular side effects.
Autonomy	Freedom to make choices and decisions independently
Care Plan	An individualised plan detailing treatment and care needs
Continuity of Care	Care offered as a continuous series of contacts over time (longitudinal continuity) from a range of service providers (cross-sectional continuity).
Day Centre	A day centre provides social care for service users and it may also offer treatment. Rehabilitation and activation services may be provided and may include occupational therapy, social skills training and light industrial therapy.
Day Hospital	A day hospital provides comprehensive treatment equivalent to that available in a hospital inpatient setting for acutely ill service users. A range of assessment and investigative procedures and treatments is carried out. The day hospital acts as the focus of psychiatric care in an area and is primarily for active treatment of patients with psychiatric disorders.
DON	Director of Nursing
GAF	General Assessment of Functioning
GP	General Practitioner
HAIL	Housing Association for Integrated Living
HoNOS	Health of the Nation Outcome Scale
HRB	Health Research Board
HSE	Health Service Executive
HSE Administrative Areas	In 2005, four new HSE administrative areas replaced the former health board areas. Within the four administrative areas there are local health office areas that correspond, in the main, to county catchment areas.
Key Worker	A staff member who usually has the most one-to-one contact with the mental health service user with complex needs. The key worker communicates with others involved in the care of the service user.
Long-stay	Continuous hospitalisation for over one year.
MHC	Mental Health Commission
NPIRS	National Psychiatric Inpatient Reporting System
Policy	A plan of action that governs mental health service activity and which employees are expected to follow.
Protocol	A written plan specifying the procedures to be followed in providing care in defined situations (Protocols specify who does what, when and how).
Planning for the Future	Title of the report of a study group on the planning of the psychiatric services. December 1984.
Skill Mix	The blend of skills needed amongst a team of staff to ensure effective health care delivery.
STEER	A community based user-led mental health organisation. Support – Training – Education – Employment – Research.
A Vision for Change	Title of the report of an expert group, which sets out a comprehensive policy framework for mental health services (2006)

Acknowledgments

The authors would like to thank the staff of the HSE local areas who contributed to this study, especially the clinical directors, directors of nursing and assistant directors of nursing and administrators. But, above all, the authors would like to thank the residents for giving so willingly of their time to participate in this project, for welcoming the researcher (DTD) into their homes and for their honesty and openness. Without their co-operation this project would not have been possible.

We would also like to thank the advisory committee for their advice and assistance throughout the study period. The advisory committee members were:

Bríd Clarke, Mental Health Commission

Fiona Keogh, Mental Health Commission

Derek Griffin, Northern Area

Pat Brosnan, Mid West Area

John Hayes, North West Area

Rhona Jennings, Mental Health Commission

Bernadette McCabe, St Vincent's Hospital, Fairview

Diarmuid Ring, Mental Health Commission

Mike Watts, Mental Health Commission

Thanks also to colleagues in the Health Research Board for providing assistance during the study period. A special thanks to Yulia Kartalova O'Doherty for her invaluable input throughout the study.

Finally the authors would like to thank the external reviewers, Mr John Saunders and Dr Sinead McGilloway, for their time and invaluable comments.

Funding from the Health Research Board and the Mental Health Commission supported this project.

Foreword

Significant changes have occurred in the profile of mental health service provision in Ireland during the last 25 years. The number and composition of community residences have grown considerably. This has had an immediate effect on reducing the number of long-stay patients in hospital as advocated in Planning for the Future (1984). In 1984, there were 121 community residences, with nine hundred (900) places. Twenty years later in 2004, the number of people living in community residences exceeded three thousand (3,065). Community residences are, therefore, now a very important element of mental health services provision in Ireland, shaping the lives of over three thousand (3,000) people and utilising considerable personnel and financial resources.

The Mental Health Commission considered it opportune to review and evaluate the role of community residences in Ireland and to report on how the needs of residents were being met and whether the community residences were fulfilling the original mandate of providing a therapeutic and rehabilitation function. The study was undertaken by the Health Research Board and jointly funded by the Mental Health Commission and Health Research Board. The information and knowledge from this study will complement the inspections of 24 hour nurse supervised community residences undertaken by the Inspectorate of Mental Health Services in 2005 and reported in detail in the Annual Report of the Mental Health Commission, including the Report of the Inspector of Mental Health Services 2005.

Research provides new knowledge and understanding and enhances strategic planning and service delivery. This study of community residences provides valuable information and evaluation of this key aspect of mental health services in Ireland. The most important component of this study is the input of the residents, who, as the prime reporting agents, expressed their views of their lives and their degree of satisfaction with current service provision.

We hope this study will inform the current philosophy and operation of community residences and future mental health service planning. Issues raised include increasing autonomy and independence of residents, promoting growth and choice, creating "a way of living a satisfying, hopeful and contributing life even with the limitations caused by illness" (Anthony 1993). Of wider social and economic significance the study supports mainstreaming housing provision for people with mental health difficulties and mainstreaming training and employment opportunities.

With the closure of mental hospitals, financial resources will become available for the development of community-based services. It is imperative that the recommendations of this report are now incorporated in development plans for mental health services.

I would like, on behalf of the Mental Health Commission, to thank all those involved in this study, the Health Research Board, the staff from the three Health Service Executive areas and the advisory committee. I wish to express my deepest appreciation to the residents who participated in this study and who shared their experiences and views with us.

Bríd Clarke
Chief Executive Officer

Mental Health Commission

January 2007

List of tables and figures

LIST OF TABLES

LIST OF FIGURES

Executive Summary

Substantial change has taken place in the mental health services in Ireland following the publication of *Planning for the Future* in 1984. That policy document recommended an accelerated move towards the provision of care in community settings and the closure of all large psychiatric hospitals. Patients with persistent mental health problems were to be relocated to alternative accommodation in community residences. The rationale was that community residences would fulfil a therapeutic and rehabilitation function such that persons with persistent mental illness would move from higher to lower levels of support, and where possible, to complete independence. The more recent mental health policy *A Vision for Change* (Department of Health and Children, 2006), emphasises the importance of independence and recovery for those with persistent mental health problems. However, there is little information in the policy about the role of community residences, a key component of community mental health provision – in providing for residents' wellbeing and independence. The present study examines the role and functions of community residences and, in particular, the extent to which they have fulfilled the expectation of *Planning for the Future* (1984) in fostering rehabilitation and independence. The study details the characteristics of the residents and the residents' perceptions of their lives in the residences. The findings inform recommendations regarding the future development and reorientation of this service component.

The study describes and evaluates the nature and quality of community residential accommodation and the extent to which it met the needs of residents. The functioning of community residences with reference to the appropriateness of premises and their operational role in providing for the residents is discussed. Residents themselves were the prime reporting agents as to the view of their lives and their degree of satisfaction with current service provision. The interaction of the residents with their neighbourhood and environment was also investigated. Enquiry was made as to their 'citizenisation', such as voting registration, participation in social amenities and use of community services. In addition, staff understanding of the aims and functions of the residences and their perceptions of the factors that promoted or impeded independent living were investigated.

STUDY FINDINGS

Three HSE local mental health service areas took part in the study – North West, Mid West and Northern Area, comprising eight catchment areas. One of these catchment areas had no community residences. There was a total of 102 residences in these areas, providing 951 places. The majority of these places were high support (584), with 166 medium support places and 201 low support places. At the time of the study there were 871 residents living in the residences, an occupancy rate of 92%. However, 76 places were designated for other uses (such as respite care), resulting in an occupancy rate of 97%.

A total of 138 residents were interviewed for the study. Of these, 59% were from high support, 18% from medium support and 22% from low support residences. Their average age was 53 years (SD 13.4), the majority were single and almost half had second level education. A large proportion of the sample were unemployed (40%), while 27% were in sheltered employment and 7% in either part-time or full-time paid employment. The residents interviewed had a long duration of illness and the majority had a diagnosis of schizophrenia.

The clinical functioning of the residents suggested that the majority had mild but stable symptoms. Their general occupational and social functioning was better in medium and low support than in high support; however, all group ratings were above the level that indicates a marked degree of disability. In general, no problems in social functioning two weeks prior to interview was reported, but mild to moderate difficulties were reported for activities of daily living. The majority of the residents were not experiencing physical health problems. Thus, the residents had a low rate of clinical symptoms, generally had good physical health and showed no marked disabilities in occupational and social functioning. The findings suggest that some residents were over-provided for in terms of the level of accommodation in which they were living.

The results of the interviews showed that, in general, the residents were satisfied with their treatment and care and their current accommodation; however a number of residents indicated that, if given a choice, they would prefer more independent living arrangements. The perceptions of the residents regarding life in the residences were mostly positive and residents reported that they had control over their lives and were happy with their level of independence.

While the majority of the residents went out on their own and reported that they were happy with their level of participation in the community, few used social amenities in the community. A large proportion of residents received staff help to mange their finances. Almost a quarter were reported to have no system of support outside the residences, while over half had visits from family and friends or made visits to family and friends. The residents themselves reported that they would rely on staff or other residents for support during a crisis, but that they would use supports from outside the residences for everyday psychological support, if available.

Among staff, the most commonly perceived functions of the residences were those of continuing care and rehabilitation. In terms of rehabilitation, the majority of residences were reported as providing a range of therapeutic activities, mainly social skills training and everyday living skills training. Fewer residences were providing cognitive behavioural therapies or activities that promoted community integration, mainstream employment or mainstream housing. This is not surprising given the lack of specialised multi-disciplinary rehabilitation teams in the services studied.

The internal environment of the residences was not ideal, with a small number of bathrooms and many shared bedrooms. Results indicate that lack of privacy was an issue for a number of residents. In general, there was good access to facilities such as shops, post offices and GP surgeries in the external environment. However, few residents had access to their own transport, which was problematic for those in more remote locations where public transport was often underdeveloped.

The climate and culture of the residences reflected more those of a 'mini-institution' than of a home-like environment, especially in the high support residences. The medium and low support residences were somewhat more relaxed, but a large number employed constricting rules and regulations, the necessity for which was questionable. There appeared to be little in the way of individualised treatment and care

planning in many of the residences, nor was there much participation by the residents in their treatment and care. The results suggested that the philosophy of a 'recovery' model was still far from realisation in these community residences. There was very close interaction between the residents and staff, and residents reported in the majority of cases that staff and residents got on very well together. However, there was evidence of an excess of care in some cases, for example the restrictive nature of residential facilities and the lack of autonomy of the residents given their current level of functioning. This most likely stemmed from the fact that many staff were trained in the care philosophy of the old psychiatric hospitals.

STUDY IMPLICATIONS

The study has provided a view of the community residence service component in the round and, most importantly, through the eyes of those who live in community residences. The findings show that there is a high level of satisfaction among residents in relation to their treatment and care and the accommodation provided. Many suggestions for improvement also emerged, which are presented in the recommendations below. But what of the service into the future and the needs of future residents? The study recommendations address the future of this community residence service component as the programme of deinstitutionalisation comes to an end and the services move towards a 'recovery' approach, whereby individuals are empowered to take more control of their own lives and participate more fully in society. This contextualisation calls into question many aspects of the role and function of community residences. These include issues such as the responsibility for the provision of residences, the internal and external environment of the residences, the climate and culture within the residences, and rehabilitation and recovery philosophies of care.

The recommendations below have been made in the light of the study findings and have taken into consideration recent policy documents and evidence-based practice. The authors were mindful of the feasibility of implementing the recommendations within the Irish mental health services and were of the opinion that the recommendations should be addressed in the short to medium term. It is the authors' intention however, that these recommendations will be evaluated in light of local area needs, requirements and resources and adapted and implemented accordingly.

STUDY RECOMMENDATIONS

Recommendations are made under four main headings – the way forward for rehabilitation and recovery, the way forward for current community residences, future provision of housing and the implementation action plan.

A summary of the recommendations are presented in the following section under the four main headings. Readers are advised to note the full list of recommendations in Chapter 11.

THE WAY FORWARD FOR REHABILITATION AND RECOVERY

- Fully staffed specialised rehabilitation and recovery mental health teams should be established in all services as a matter of urgency.

- All members of the specialised rehabilitation team should be trained in the competencies and principles of recovery.

- All current and potential residents should receive a full multidisciplinary assessment.

- Staff should, by attitude and practice, orient residents towards raising their expectations of their capabilities to achieve independence.

- Individual care plans should be developed with residents and should incorporate their expectations and be reviewed on a regular basis.

- A key worker system should be in place in all areas.

- The pharmacological treatment of residents should be reviewed regularly, especially those on multiple medications.

- Rehabilitative activities should be tailored to meet the needs of the individual.

- The possibility of moving rehabilitative activities to the community and availing of existing community-based activities should be explored and developed.

- Residents should be encouraged and provided with the necessary skills to look after their own finances.

- Residents should be encouraged to develop and extend social support networks.

- Mainstream employment using the 'place and train' model coupled with other employment and training initiatives should be developed with the relevant stakeholders and evaluated.

THE WAY FORWARD FOR CURRENT RESIDENCES

- Community residences should be used only for support and rehabilitation.

- All staff should be trained in the competencies necessary to provide a recovery-oriented service.

- Residences should provide a 'home-like' environment for residents.

- The number of places in high support residences should be reduced to ten.

- Nursing resources currently employed in community residences should be evaluated and the proper skill mix of staff ensured.

- Evaluation and review plans should be implemented in the residences to monitor quality, including residents' satisfaction.

- Aims and functions of community residences should be reviewed and standardised.

FUTURE PROVISION OF HOUSING

- Housing for those with mental health difficulties must be provided as part of mainstream housing and is not the responsibility of the mental health services.

- The provision of low and medium support housing should be the responsibility of the local housing authorities.

- A range of housing alternatives is necessary to meet the needs and support requirements of individuals with different mental health needs.

☐ Multi-agency groups involving, among others, local housing authorities and mental health service providers, should be set up as a matter of urgency to discuss partnership schemes in the provision of housing and care.

☐ Pilot schemes for the provision of housing that have been shown to be effective should be encouraged and should receive financial support.

☐ All future housing should be designed with the principles of recovery in mind.

IMPLEMENTATION ACTION PLAN

☐ The study recommendations must be implemented without delay.

☐ Intersectoral action plans must be formulated at central and local level and must represent housing and mental health interests.

☐ The local group will report on progress to the central group.

☐ An intersectoral implementation group should be formed at central level. This group should lead on intersectoral policy changes required, monitor progress towards implementation and liaise with the implementation and monitoring bodies of *A Vision for Change*.

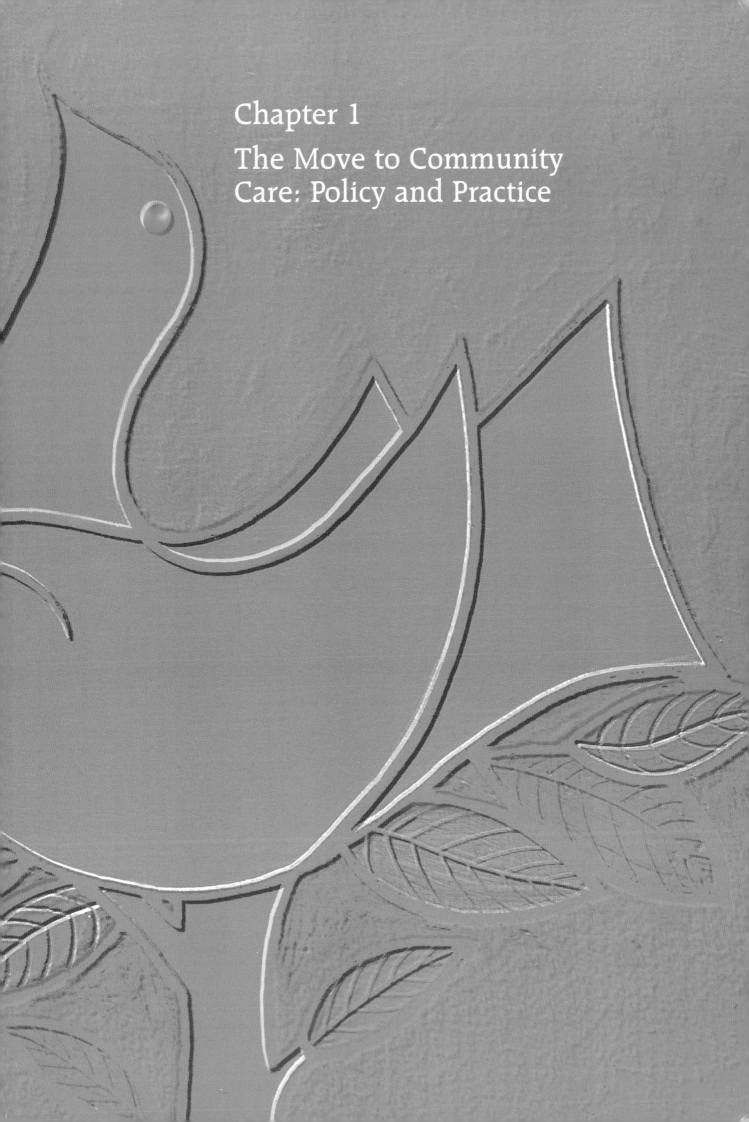

Chapter 1
The Move to Community
Care: Policy and Practice

CHAPTER 1

The move to community care: policy and practice

1.1 INTRODUCTION

It is estimated that 450 million people worldwide suffer from mental health problems (World Health Organization (WHO), 2003). Furthermore, it is estimated that mental health problems will increase from 12% of the total burden of disease to 15% by 2020. This confirms psychiatric disorder as one of the leading causes of disease and disability. WHO estimates that one in four people visiting a health service has mental health difficulties that are often undiagnosed and untreated. WHO reports that cost-effective treatments do exist for most mental health problems and, if appropriately used, could result in enabling most individuals to become fully functioning members of society.

Irish mental health polices, such as *Planning for the Future*, have emphasised the closing of psychiatric hospitals and substituting institutional care with care in the community (Department of Health and Children, 1984). In the last twenty years a substantial change has taken place in the Irish mental health services. The programme of deinstitutionalisation has accelerated in most areas and, while this is not yet complete, many individuals have been relocated to community-based residences. A recent development has been the publication of *A Vision for Change* (2006), which outlines the continued developments necessary for mental health services to meet evidence-based standards of practice and care and to ensure that the fundamental rights of mental heath service users are met.

Among the recommendations for community care was the provision of community residential facilities for the relocation of long-stay patients from psychiatric hospitals. The rationale was that these community residences should fulfil a therapeutic and rehabilitation function such that residents passed from higher levels of dependency to lower levels of support and, where possible, to complete independence. No previous research in Ireland has investigated the quality of the mental health services community residences and the extent to which the services meet the needs of the residents.

This study aimed to describe and evaluate the nature and quality of community residential accommodation in a sample of three HSE local areas in Ireland and the extent to which this provision has accomplished the policy objective (more information on the aims and objectives of the study are presented in Chapter 2). The three participating HSE local areas were the North West Area, the Mid West Area and the Northern Area. The North West includes the catchment areas of Donegal and Sligo. The Mid West comprises the catchment areas of Limerick, Clare and North Tipperary. The Northern Area includes the catchment areas of Dublin North West (Mental Health Area 6), Dublin North City (Mental Health Area 7) and Dublin North (Mental Health Area 8). These areas are located within two HSE administrative areas. The North West and the Mid West are located in HSE administrative area A, while the HSE administrative area B includes the Northern Area. More information on the participating areas is presented in Chapter 3.

Although there have been some surveys of the extent of mental illness in specific population groups, such as the elderly (Shiely & Kelleher, 2004; McGee *et al.*, 2005) no comprehensive community-based data exist on psychiatric morbidity in the general adult population in Ireland. Data from a pilot study suggest that 25% of patients attending general practice in Ireland have mental health problems (Copty & Whitford, 2005). The majority of these (95%) are dealt with in primary care with the rest being referred to mental health services. The Mental Health Research Division (MHRD) of the Health Research Board (HRB) is currently carrying out a survey to assess psychological distress, service use and help-seeking behaviour in the general population. This survey should help to bridge the current information gap in terms of assessing the level of psychological distress in the population and mental health service needs.

There is some indication of the mental health service activity levels at secondary-level care. The Medico-Social Research Board, later to be amalgamated with the

Medical Research Council (MRC) to become the Health Research Board (HRB), has been collecting statistics on activity at inpatient psychiatric hospitals and units for almost forty years. The latest figures (Daly et al., 2005) show that there were 22,279 admissions to psychiatric hospitals and units in Ireland during 2004, resulting in a rate of 735 admissions for every 100,000 persons aged 16 years and over. It is important to note that these figures represent all admissions – first admissions and re-admissions. In the absence of an individual patient identifier, it is not possible to determine how many individual patients are represented in the re-admission figures.[1] First admissions, on the other hand, refer to unique individuals and there were 6,134 first admissions in 2004 – a rate of 202 per 100,000 persons aged 16 and over. These national inpatient data are reported on by age, gender and other variables in annual reports from National Psychiatric Inpatient Recording System (NPIRS).

While the inpatient activity of mental health services has been recorded and reported on, there is a lack of information concerning activity within other components of the mental health service. This is of particular concern in the current time of change and the move towards a community based service. The HRB has developed a database, COMCAR, to record activity at community care level. This database is currently being piloted in numerous sites around the country, prior to national roll-out. It is important to note that the absence of mental health information systems has been highlighted in the Report of the Inspector of Mental Health Services (MHC, 2005a) which states that information 'is fundamental to the delivery and management of any business or service'. The HRB and MHC have set up a committee to devise a minimum data set for mental health services.

Concerning our capacity to respond to problems of mental illness and the under-funding of the mental health services, the Report of the Inspector of Mental Health Services (MHC, 2005a) highlighted the under-funding of the mental health services, which in 2004 was 7% of

national health expenditure. The Report argues that an increase of 5% bringing expenditure to 12% of the national health budget, is required. This is in line with the estimates of mental health problems accounting for 12% of the total burden of disease and with proportional mental health expenditure in the United Kingdom.

1.2 POLICY FRAMEWORK: THE MOVE FROM INSTITUTIONAL CARE

Prior to the mid-eighteenth century, mental illness was not a major social concern and was often viewed as the consequence of 'possession' and witchcraft. It aroused bewilderment and confusion and was often dealt with harshly and punitively. A century later, the problem of mental ill health had increased to such an extent that a national system of lunatic asylums was established in Ireland. This reflected the national policy of institutionalisation of the mentally ill in Ireland as elsewhere which was to persist for almost a century and a half.

In Ireland, the 1945 Mental Treatment Act allowed for the 'boarding out' of detained patients and for voluntary admission to district psychiatric hospitals. However, admissions to inpatient care continued to increase and the 'boarding out' of patients was not adopted on a national level. Institutionalisation reached its peak in Ireland in 1958 when over 21,000 persons were resident in our psychiatric hospitals, about 3,000 of whom were intellectually disabled.

With the growth in provision of alternative forms of care, such as outpatient clinics, and the introduction of antipsychotic and antidepressant drugs, coupled with concern about the conditions in psychiatric hospitals and a growing civil rights movement, the numbers of those detained for long periods in psychiatric hospitals declined. These improvements, which had begun in other jurisdictions, spread to Ireland, where existing conditions were sharply critised and the need to move to community care for the mentally ill was emphasised by the *Report of the*

Commission of Enquiry on Mental Illness in 1966. The recommendations of the Commission were reinforced by another national policy document in the field of mental health, *Planning for the Future,* in 1984.

Policy documents and legalistic provisions fundamental to the development and change in mental health services in Ireland have included *Planning for the Future* (1984) and the Mental Health Act (2001). More recently a new policy document, *A Vision for Change* (2006), provided a policy framework for the development of mental health services for the next seven to ten years.

1.2.1 The community residential alternative to long-stay hospitalisation

The 1966 Commission recommended that the number of hospitalisations should be reduced by 1981. However, the recommendations relating to community placement of the long-stay inpatient was meagrely implemented, so that by 1981 the numbers hospitalised still stood at 15,000 rather than the 8,000 that the Commission had visualised. *Planning for the Future* (1984) specifically addressed this particular problem.

That report argued for a comprehensive mental health service to provide care for the varying needs of people with mental health problems. This service was to include community-based residences to which suitable long-stay patients from the psychiatric hospitals could be relocated. The report proposed four categories of persons who would be more suitably placed in the community residential services, as follows:

☐ Persons now living in psychiatric hospitals who have no homes of their own to return to but who, with adequate preparation and training, would be capable of living a reasonable life in the community;

☐ Persons coming forward for psychiatric care with chronic psychiatric disability, who have inadequate or no homes and who would be capable of living with varying degrees of independence in accommodation in the community;

☐ Persons with psychiatric problems whose treatment requires that they live apart from their family or normal associates for a while – such persons include disturbed teenagers who have family difficulties and patients in need of temporary accommodation due to any of a variety of social reasons;

☐ The small group of new long stay patients for whom high support hostels will provide an alternative to long-stay hospital care. (Department of Health and Children, 1984: p.60)

In 1989 the priorities for the future development of the mental health services were outlined in the document *Shaping a Healthier Future* (Department of Health and Children, 1989). These included the establishment of departments of psychiatry in general hospitals and the introduction of a new Mental Health Act which would, inter alia, meet the requirements of the European Convention on Human Rights. A White Paper (Department of Health and Children, 1995) reaffirmed the need for the protection of patients admitted involuntarily and further highlighted the need for new legislation.

1.2.2 Mental Health Act 2001

The Mental Health Act of 2001 proposes significant changes to certain aspects of the mental health services in Ireland. It is concerned with the involuntary admission of persons in psychiatric hospitals, the monitoring and evaluation of

1   Local figures from the Mid West suggested that, on average, each person accounted for 2.5 admissions.

approved centres, mental health services, and the legal rights of psychiatric patients. It also provides the legislative basis for the establishment of the Mental Health Commission (MHC) – an independent body with responsibility to promote good practice and high standards in the delivery of mental health services and to protect the interest of people admitted involuntarily to psychiatric hospitals and units. The MHC in its Strategic Plan 2004–2005, highlighted and supported the notion of community care in place of inpatient care. The MHC has also stimulated the debate on mental health service provision and quality with the publication of three discussion papers. These are: *A Vision for a Recovery Model in Irish Mental Health Services* (MHC, 2005b), *Multidisciplinary Team Working: From Theory to Practice* (MHC, 2006a) and *Forensic Mental Health Services for Adults in Ireland* (MHC, 2006b). The MHC also commissioned a research study investigating service users' and stakeholders' perceptions of quality in mental health services (MHC, 2005c). A recent report commissioned by the MHC showed that the organisation of public mental health services was inappropriate and unsuited to the needs of those who use these services (Dunne, 2006). This is an important step in using research and service users' and stakeholder input to inform practice and policy.

The Mental Health Act 2001 provides for the appointment of an Inspector of Mental Health Services in place of the previous post of Inspector of Mental Hospitals. The Inspector of Mental Health Services has responsibility for the inspection of all approved inpatient centres and other centres where mental health services are provided. In addition, the inspectorate ascertains the service users' and carers' views on their local services. This information facilitates the Mental Health

Commission's statutory responsibility to 'promote, encourage and foster the establishment and maintenance of high standards and good practice in the delivery of mental health services'. The Inspectorate's first full report was published in 2005 (MHC, 2005a). This report highlighted that, although the living conditions of many people were improved by the relocation from the long stay wards in hospitals to community residences, without specialist rehabilitative input 'such residences became little better than long-stay wards in a community setting'. The Inspector also pointed out that 35 rehabilitation teams were required nationally. The provision of this specialised care and support should result in a decrease in the number of psychiatric beds as long-stay patients are moved to the community, in addition to a reduction in 24-hour staffed community placements as those newly presenting with severe mental illness are provided with care and support to live independently in the community (MHC, 2005a).

1.2.3 A Vision for Change

The most recent document concerning policy in mental health services in Ireland is the report, *A Vision for Change,* by the Expert Group on Mental Health Policy (Department of Health and Children, 2006). It details recommendations on how the mental health services in Ireland should develop over the next seven to ten years. A phased development is recommended which should be in line with the reorganisation of the mental health services in the new health service structures. The document proposes a policy framework that adopts a lifespan approach to mental health. It covers all areas of mental health service provision from primary care to specialist care. The Report emphasises a community-based approach with inpatient services used sparingly. It takes a holistic view of mental health that addresses biological, psychological and social factors and consequently advocates a multidisciplinary approach. The Report was devised in consultation with service users, carers, providers and other stakeholders and covered all aspects of the service from evidence-based interventions to the management and the financing of the services. *A Vision for Change* sees service users' and carers' views as critical to the development and planning of services. In addition, the Report recommends the importance of empowering service users to take responsibility for their care in partnership with providers. This document clearly sets the scene for the future development of the mental health services which are without doubt firmly placed within a community-care model.

In relation to the issue of providing for the recovery and rehabilitation of persons with severe and persistent illness, *A Vision for Change* envisioned that the housing for persons with or recovering from mental illness would be supplied by local housing authorities in routine, normal houses which would be in no different from those available to other clients housed by them. The Report recommended three residential units of 10 places each per 100,000 population for those whose enduring problems would be of such intensity that a high level of support by the mental health services would be required. It is envisaged that, once the cohort of existing long-stay patients has been accommodated, the requirement for high support accommodation will decline. Thus, the main housing requirement into the future will be for individualised, independent accommodation with some support, as appropriate, from the mental health services working co-operatively with the housing authorities. It is pointed out unambiguously that the statutory responsibility for housing lies

squarely with the housing authorities and should not be within the remit of the mental health services. The Report points out that a considerable deviation of mental health resources has resulted from the practice of mental health services providing accommodation which is statutorily the responsibility of housing authorities. The Report further alludes to the necessity of using housing in a flexible progressive fashion to best accommodate the changing needs of patients as recovery proceeds. It is felt that crisis housing accommodation would best be accomplished by special crisis units on the basis of one per region of 300,000. It was argued that the current practise of designating a number of beds in routine mental health housing for this purpose, and that such mixing of patients, aims and purposes was not in the best interests of either group.

1.2.4 European framework for mental health

The World Health Organization (WHO) European office has developed a *Mental Health Declaration for Europe* (2005) and an accompanying *Mental Health Action Plan for Europe* (2005). These have been endorsed by Ministers from the European WHO member states (January 2005). These documents proposed the priorities for mental health over the next 10 years and specified actions to meet these priorities. The following five priorities were listed in the Declaration:

☐ Foster an awareness of mental health.

☐ Tackle stigma, discrimination and inequality and empower those with mental health problems and their families to engage in this process.

☐ Design and implement comprehensive mental health

Figure 1.1   Provision of community residential places in Ireland for five-year intervals from 1983 to 2003

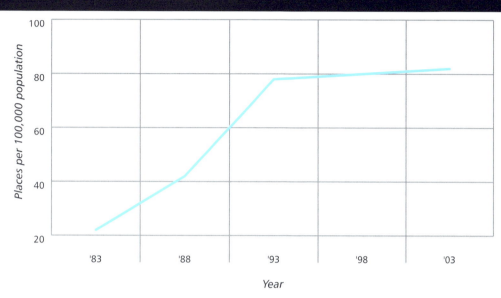

systems that cover mental health promotion, prevention, treatment and rehabilitation and care and recovery.

☐ Create a competent workforce with the necessary skills for effective treatment and care in all areas.

☐ Recognise the experience of the user and the families and carers and the importance of this experience for service planning and development

The WHO Action Plan presented a number of actions under twelve headings, which ranged from mental health promotion, treatment and care, evaluation of effectiveness and funding of mental health services. Regarding the location of mental health services, the plan advocated that provision should be firmly placed within the community, with a limited number of hospital beds. The document recognised the importance of a comprehensive multidisciplinary service that empowers service users to work in partnership with service providers. Actions to address stigma and

discrimination were proposed as were actions to establish partnership across sectors. It is envisaged that the member states of the WHO European Region will use the actions laid out in the Action Plan to develop and implement comprehensive policies in their countries. The recently published EU Green Paper aimed at the development of an EU strategy on mental health articulates similar themes (Commission of the European Communities, 2005). The recommendations of Irish policy documents, especially those reported in *A Vision for Change* are in line with current European thinking in the area.

1.3 FROM POLICY TO PRACTICE: COMMUNITY RESIDENTIAL CARE IN IRELAND

The move in policy and practice to community care in Ireland resulted in a decline in the overall number of inpatients in psychiatric hospitals and units and an increase in the number of community residential facilities as patients were relocated to the community. As a result of the implementation of this policy, the number of persons in inpatient care had declined to 3,389 persons by the end of March 2006 (Daly & Walsh, 2006). Of these, 997 were long-stay in hospital (i.e. in hospital for more than five years) and 548 were categorised as 'new long-stay' (i.e. in hospital for more than one but less than five years).

The figures for community residential facilities in Ireland were reported in the *Report of the Inspectorate of Mental Hospitals* until 2003 when there was inter-organisational shift in the responsibility for producing the report of the mental health services. Figure 1.1 shows the total number of community residential places per 100, 000 population for five-year intervals from 1983 to 2003. Figures for the number of residents in community residential facilities in 2004 were provided by the Mental Health Commission (MHC, personal communication).

There was a total of 111 community residential facilities in Ireland in 1983, 233 in 1988, 361 in 1993, 386 in 1998 and 418 in 2003. Thus, the number of residences doubled between 1983 and 1988 following the publication of *Planning for the Future* (1984). This increase continued to 2003, although at a slower rate. The facilities provided 942 places in 1983, which increased to 3,210 in 2003. The corresponding rates were 27 places per 100, 000 population in 1983 and 82 per 100, 000 population in 2003 (Figure 1.1). As in the number of facilities, the largest increase in rate of places per 100, 000 occurred following the publication of *Planning for the Future* in 1984 and continued during the period 1988 to 1993. The most recent figures in 2004 reported there were 3,065 residents living in the community residential facilities, a rate of 101.2 residents per 100,000 population aged 16 years and over (MHC, personal communication).

These figures suggest that the policy of deinstitutionalisation was indeed implemented in the eighties and early nineties and that large numbers of patients were relocated from inpatient care

to alternative community residences. There are now approximately 1,755 patients in public psychiatric hospitals – 774 being long-stay patients, of whom 408 are aged over 65 years (Daly & Walsh, 2006). As reviewed above, recent Irish policy advocated that the remaining psychiatric hospitals be closed and patients moved to community care (MHC 2005a; MHC 2006c).

1.4   STRUCTURE OF ADULT MENTAL HEALTH SERVICES IN IRELAND

Until 2005 the health services in Ireland were organised and managed by statutory bodies (health boards) and were based on geographical regions. These health boards were responsible for the health and social services of the population within the designated boundaries. In 2004, the health service delivery system was restructured by legislation. A new body was established, the Health Service Executive (HSE), which resulted in the dissolution of the old health board areas. In addition to taking over the roles and responsibilities of the previous health boards, the HSE is tasked with developing services in line with the most recent health strategy, *Quality and Fairness: A Health System for You* (Department of Health and Children, 2001), such as the inclusion of service users in decision making and service planning. Changes to the organisation of the health service came into effect in January 2005, with Health Service Executive administrative regions and local areas replacing health board areas. Where there were eight health board areas, there are now four HSE administrative areas with populations of approximately 1,000,000 each. The local health office areas within these areas correspond, in the main, to the county catchment areas.

Suggestions as to the best way forward for the delivery of mental health services within the new health service structure was reported in *A Vision for Change*. It was argued that the existing small catchment areas of about 100, 000 population have hindered the development of specialised mental health services (Inspector of Mental Health Services, Mental Health Commission, 2005a). *A Vision for Change* reported that catchment areas should be increased in size from approximately 100,000 population to between 200,000 and 400,000. Catchment area size will depend on the characteristics of the population and on geographical factors. The larger catchment areas will allow for the inclusion of specialised mental health services in areas that are accessible to the population. *A Vision for Change* proposed that sectorisation remain and that sector size be increased from 25,000 to 50,000. To date, no major changes have occurred in the management or delivery of the mental health services since the changes in the health service structures. Following the recommendations in *A Vision for Change,* an implementation review committee was established to ensure the implementation and evaluation of the recommendations within the seven to ten year time span.

1.5 SUMMARY

The recommendation to move from institutional to community care has been reiterated in many national and international policy documents over the past 40 years. The relocation of patients from large institutions in Ireland has been slow and variable across the country and there are now approximately 15 old-style psychiatric hospitals still in operation. While inpatient beds have been reduced as the availability of community residential places increased, no research has been conducted to evaluate the utility and function of these residential facilities on a national level. While there has been local research to review community accommodation, for example within the mental health services in the Northern Area (Health Service Executive, 2004) and in the North West area (The Sainsbury Centre for Mental Health, 2004), there is little indication of the degree to which the residents are satisfied with treatment and care and other aspects of their lives or the extent of their autonomy.

CHAPTER 2
Rehabilitation and Recovery: An Overview

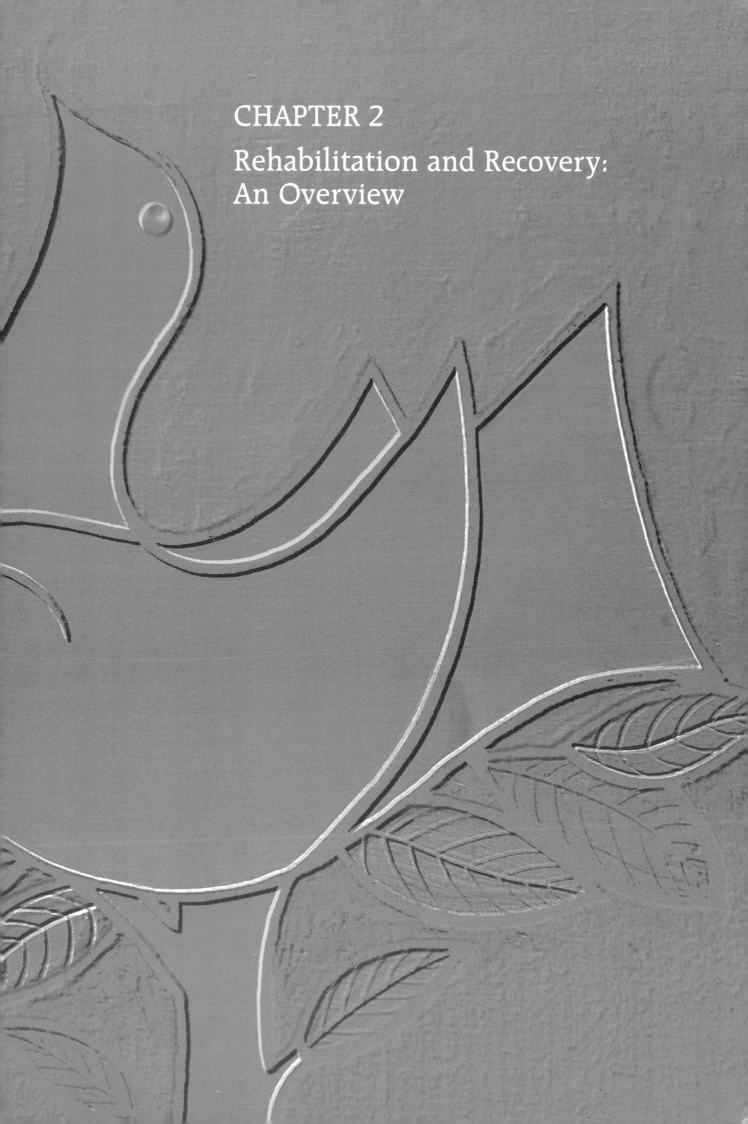

Chapter 2

Rehabilitation and recovery: an overview

2.1 INTRODUCTION

The following sections provide a brief overview of the literature relevant to the study. Given the wide breath of the topics covered and the vast amount of empirical literature in the areas, an in-depth review of the literature was beyond the scope of the study.

Traditionally, mental health services were delivered mainly within a structured hospital setting and physical treatments and medication were the main treatments provided to patients. Very little attention was given to other aspects of the person's wellbeing in the way of addressing social or occupational disabilities or follow-up and support on hospital discharge. In fact, the culture and the atmosphere of psychiatric hospitals were thought to exacerbate and add to the problems of long-stay patients (British Psychological Society, 2000). With the movement towards community-based care, other aspects of the person's treatment and wellbeing needed consideration and this, in turn, led to the development of community psychiatry.

2.2 COMMUNITY PSYCHIATRY DEFINED

In the 1980s, following the move to community care, Tansella (1986) defined community psychiatry as

"a system of care devoted to a defined population and based on a comprehensive and integrated mental health service, which includes outpatient facilities, day and residential training centres, residential accommodation hostels, sheltered workshops and inpatient units in general hospitals, and which ensures, with multidisciplinary team-work, early diagnosis, prompt treatment, continuity of care, social support and a close liaison with other medical and social community services and, in particular, with general practitioners."

Tansella's definition thus included the social, physical and mental wellbeing of the individual. Szmukler and Thornicroft

(2001) argued that community psychiatry referred to the work not only of the medical professionals, but of all mental health professionals, including nurses, psychologists, social workers and occupational therapists. They stressed that community psychiatry should provide whatever care and treatment is necessary to meet the needs of a defined population. They argued that the three fundamental principles underlying community psychiatry were:

- ☐ Care and treatment should be provided to all in the population in relation to need.

- ☐ Evidence-based treatment should be delivered wherever necessary and such treatment should be accessible to and accepted by the patient.

- ☐ Care and treatment involve a network of elements addressing health and social care. Services required may be provided by voluntary, private or public sectors. The quality of the service will depend on the interconnectedness of these elements.

The principle of a network of elements of care is very important, especially for those with persistent symptoms, which can cause distress for the individual and their family. However, the reduction of symptoms is not necessarily sufficient to bring about an improvement in the quality of life of the individual (Mikrim & Namerow, 1991). Social, cognitive and occupational functioning can impact immensely on the quality of life and the social inclusion of the individual. Problems in functioning can occur as a direct result of the disorder or indirectly, for example as a result of the side effects of medication, stigma, institutionalisation or social exclusion. There is a need for a holistic approach to treatment and care, as opposed to the traditional medical approach.

Thornicroft and Tansella (1999) define a community mental health service as

- ☐ one which provides a full range of effective mental health care to a defined population, and which is dedicated to treating and helping people with mental disorders, in proportion to their suffering or distress, in collaboration with other local agencies.

Quality of services must be evaluated on the principles underlying community mental health care. These principles, as identified by Tansella and Thornicroft (2001), include:

☐ Autonomy – the freedom to make independent choices despite the presence of symptoms of disabilities

☐ Continuity – the ability of services to provide consistent interventions at the patient level or at the local level

☐ Effectiveness – proven interventions offered to patients

☐ Accessibility – the ability of the services to provide care when and where required

☐ Comprehensiveness – the ability of services to provide treatment and care across a range of severities and patient characteristics

☐ Equity – the fair allocation of resources for services, based on needs assessment.

☐ Accountability – the ability of services to meet the expectations of the patient, families and the wider public

☐ Co-ordination – the ability of services to provide a coherent treatment plan for patients that include clear goals and interventions that are needed and effective. Services should be co-ordinated within an episode of care and between agencies

☐ Efficiency – the ability of services to provide economic efficiency by minimising the costs of inputs to achieve required outcomes or by increasing the effectiveness or quality of outcomes on a fixed budget.

More recently, Thornicroft and Tansella (2004) argued for a balanced approach to mental health service provision that includes both modern hospital-based care and modern community-based care. The balanced-care approach focuses on providing services in community settings and prompt admission to hospital-based care only when necessary. Care in the community should be provided as close as possible to the population served.

2.3   PSYCHIATRIC REHABILITATION

Concepts of community psychiatry and community-based care highlighted the need for services that were traditionally based within the hospital to move to the community. Rehabilitation services for those with severe mental illness were traditionally offered within the hospital setting. The rehabilitation and teaching of skills within the artificial setting of the hospital did not readily transfer to the individual's real world on discharge (Anthony et al., 1982). Furthermore, as programmes were based in hospitals, patients had little opportunity to integrate with the local community. The programmes were not aimed at the individual's needs and requirements, rather they tended to be offered on a group basis. This resulted in maintenance programmes as opposed to programmes that empowered the individual to move to the next stage of independence. Psychiatric rehabilitation attempted to address issue.

Psychiatric rehabilitation is defined as a process that enables those who are impaired, disabled or handicapped by a mental disorder to reach their optimal level of functioning in the community (WHO, 1996). The level of functioning includes social, occupational and economic functioning and aims to help the individual achieve as independent a life as possible in these areas. Psychosocial rehabilitation aims to reduce symptomatology and the negative effects of medications, improve social competence, reduce stigma and discrimination, improve family and social support and increase consumer empowerment (WHO, 2003). Therefore, psychosocial rehabilitation should not only be concerned with the rehabilitation of an individual's psychosocial functioning, but should also address psychosocial factors at a service level such as policy and quality of care and at a societal level such as public attitudes and legislation. Interventions aimed at improving psychosocial functioning operate at the individual level. At the service level, psychosocial rehabilitation is concerned with policy, funding, staff training and quality of care. Legislation, user involvement and public attitudes and opinions occur at the societal level of operation.

A programme of rehabilitation should include medical treatments and other interventions such as vocational rehabilitation, social skills training, proven psychosocial interventions and integration into the community (Schizophrenia Ireland, 2003). The following interventions have been identified as important in the rehabilitation of the individual towards an optimal level of functioning (WHO, 1996). Individuals should be able to access these services when and as they need them.

☐ Pharmacological treatment – it is essential that appropriate medication be used for the reduction of symptoms and reducing relapse

☐ Independent living skills and social skills training – these are most beneficial when offered in a real everyday setting

☐ Psychological support to patients and their families – this includes psychological interventions aimed at providing support and education to service users and their families. It also involves the provision of information regarding rights and the availability of psychosocial resources

☐ Vocational rehabilitation and employment – the importance of employment and training is emphasised. Training must be provided in a real-world context. Employment can take the form of sheltered employment or supported employment in the competitive job market. Supported work projects with organisations have become the preferred model of employment within the UK (Royal College of Psychiatrists, 2003)

☐ Social support networks – social support has a positive role in the mental health of an individual in strengthening the ability to cope. Individuals should be supported and encouraged to develop a social support network

☐ Leisure – all individuals must have the opportunity to participate and enjoy leisure activities of their own choice. Access to activities and freedom of choice are essential.

Effective rehabilitation will involve medical and other professionals. The current recommendation for staffing of an adult mental health rehabilitation service team includes a psychiatrist, mental health nurses, mental health support workers, occupational therapists, social workers, clinical psychologists, cognitive behaviour therapists, addiction counsellors, skill training staff, administration and staff for day centres and community residences (A Vision for Change). There is a need for the rehabilitation and recovery mental health team to work closely with other statutory health and social services and voluntary groups. For example, unmet housing and employment needs can cause immense difficulties for those with severe mental health problems. Close liaison of the rehabilitation and recovery mental health team with services that have a statutory responsibility in these areas is of great importance to the individual's recovery.

The Royal College of Psychiatrists (2003) pointed out that rehabilitation services must address issues of access to welfare rights and advocacy. There should be a detailed assessment which includes clinical, physical and social functioning, user and carer aspirations, psychiatric history, and risk assessment and management. From this assessment an individual care plan should be drawn up and a key worker assigned to the individual. Assessments should involve the individual and in some cases, with the consent of the individual, a relative or advocate (Schizophrenia Ireland, 2003). Components of the rehabilitation programme should be accessed when they are needed and the interventions should be detailed in the care plan. Needs should be regularly reviewed and the care plan amended as necessary (Department of Health, 2000).

To summarise, psychiatric rehabilitation requires a comprehensive range of medical, psychological and social therapies aimed at the needs of the service user. *A Vision for Change* recommends that multidisciplinary community mental health teams should include the 'core skills of psychiatry, nursing, social work, clinical psychology and occupational therapy'. It further argues that the principle of recovery should underlie the work of multidisciplinary rehabilitation community mental health teams. The following section elaborates on this principle.

2.4   THE SERVICE-USER MOVEMENT AND RECOVERY

There are now growing service-user movements in the UK, Ireland and elsewhere. Within Ireland the user movement is evident in Schizophrenia Ireland (SI), Support-Training-Education-Employment-Research (STEER), Mental Health Ireland (MHI) and the Irish Advocacy Network. The aims of the user movement include: to encourage self-help, to challenge assumptions about mental illness, to engage in advocacy and to campaign for improved services and to combat stigma. The user movement advocates that a sense of control over one's life is important, and holds that those who rely on services for support are often placed in a dependent position. The movement proposes that those who have experienced mental health problems have gained an expertise that can be of great benefit to others. People who have had psychotic experiences can co-educate others who have psychotic episodes, as well as mental health professionals and the public, so that these experiences can be viewed in a more positive light.

Recovery has been the topic of philosophical debate over the last 20 years and is an important concept within the service-user movement. The most widely accepted definition of recovery is that of

Anthony (1993) who said that recovery is 'a deeply personal, unique process of changing one's attitudes, values, feelings, goals skills and roles. It is a way of living a satisfying, hopeful, and contributing life even with limitations caused by illness'. The recovery approach focuses on the individual's personal path of recovery (Roberts & Wolfson, 2004) and the process by which the person adapts to living with mental health difficulties. The principle of recovery requires mutual respect across all service levels and the belief that all service users can gain control over their lives and participate fully in the community. The process of recovery is most eloquently described in personal narratives and the views of 'experts by experience' (Ralph *et al.*, 2002).

Efforts to measure recovery are still at an early stage of development. While scales have been developed to measure rehabilitation in terms of sympotomology and social functioning, no quantitative measure exists whereby the concept of recovery can be measured. The concept of recovery is a complex one and, therefore, to assess it using a single measure is difficult. The recovery approach does not dismiss the importance of medical or mental health professionals (Roberts and Wolfson, 2004; Liberman and Kopelowicz, 2005). Rather the approach sees the role of the professional as providing support by listening to the individual's life story and helping them identify necessary resources and skills training. The move to a recovery-oriented service involves a change in the role of the professional from 'expert and authority figure' to 'coach or personal trainer' (Anthony, 1993). The role of the professional is not to 'do things to people', as was in the past, but rather to listen to the individuals who are experiencing symptoms and advise them on appropriate interventions that best meet their needs. Professionals can offer skills and knowledge while at the same time listening and valuing the service user or 'expert by experience'. It is no longer acceptable that the people using mental health services remain passive users of the service (Anthony, 1993). Care providers must realise that 'each person must be in charge of and responsible for his or her own recovery' (Copeland, 2006). Copeland argues that there is a need for mental health service users to learn their rights – those that 'most people take for granted' and to 'speak out'. These include the right to choice and the right to determine what best meets their needs. It must be noted, however, that many people will have been in a service that for the most part has ignored their voices, therefore training and education in the principles of recovery are necessary.

The move to a recovery approach in mental health services has been slow, but has gathered some momentum in recent years. For example, the Royal College of Psychiatrists, (2003) in the UK emphasised the importance of the principles of recovery in redefining rehabilitation services, as did *A Vision for Change* in Ireland. *A Vision for Change* states that 'a strong commitment to the principle of "recovery" should underpin the work of the rehabilitation CMHT – the belief that it is possible for all service users to achieve control over their lives, to recover their self-esteem, and move towards building a life where they experience a sense of belonging and participation'.

A recent study on service users' views highlighted the lack of a recovery-oriented mental health service in Ireland (Schizophrenia Ireland, 2006), with service-users reporting little choice in their mental health treatment. The MHC (2005b) stimulated debate on the recovery approach in Ireland with the discussion paper *A Vision for a Recovery Model in Irish Mental Health Services*. It is envisaged that, following feedback from stakeholders, service providers and service users, a position paper on the role of the recovery approach in mental health services in Ireland will be published. This discussion paper highlighted important developments and advances in other countries for a recovery-oriented service.

In the absence of a comprehensive rehabilitation and recovery-oriented service, aspects of recovery such as employment, housing and social isolation will be neglected. The importance of a service that actively promotes and

encourages recovery and rehabilitation from mental illness cannot be over-stressed. There is a need to move away from the traditional maintenance rehabilitation model to a model that emphasises recovery, instils hope and empowerment and encourages users to gain control over their lives and achieve their own life goals. Rehabilitation services should have multiple points of access and should offer choices to service users. Rehabilitation services should emphasise a partnership between service users and service providers. The MHC in it's discussion paper highlights that the 'recovery model' in mental health services emphasises the expectation of recovery from mental ill health and promotes both enhanced self-management for service users and the development of services which facilitate the individual's personal journey towards recovery. As discussed by both the MHC discussion paper (2005b) and *A Vision for Change*, there is a need for the mental health services in Ireland to adopt a recovery-oriented approach.

2.5   SOCIAL INCLUSION

The importance of social inclusion for recovery from mental illness cannot be overstressed (Warner, 1985). Social inclusion refers to the right of the individual to participate in all areas of society and the community that they live in and to access services that are provided in that community. Unless individuals can avail of these rights, their participation in the community is limited and therefore, recovery inhibited. Social exclusion is defined as 'a series of problems that are interconnected and include poverty, discrimination, unemployment, low skills, poor housing and poor health' (Rankin, 2005a). The Irish National Action Plan against Poverty and Social Exclusion 2003–2005 is an important document that identified specific targets for addressing social exclusion in Ireland (Office for Social Inclusion, 2003).

People with mental health problems are one of the most excluded groups in society, whether they live in the hospital or the community (British Psychological Society, 2000). Those experiencing mental health problems should have the same basic rights of access to education and employment as others in society, but typically do not exercise these rights. The dependence on state benefits can often result in further exclusion from services because of poverty and other factors. A study of people attending long-term day care found that one-third did not use any recreational facilities (e.g. libraries, pubs, public leisure centres, community centres) and a small but significant percentage did not use public services such as shops, post office and public transport (Brugha *et al*, 1988). The evidence suggests that social exclusion can exacerbate clinical symptoms and social functioning and that impairments thought to be a direct result of the illness can in fact be due to social factors (British Psychological Society, 2000). Furthermore, those with mental health problems are one of the groups that have benefited least from policies that tackle disadvantage in the UK (Social Exclusion Unit, 2004). Within the Irish context, the Irish National Action Plan against Poverty and Social Inclusion 2003 – 2005, failed to identify those with mental illnesses as a vulnerable group (Office for Social Inclusion, 2003). There were no specific targets set in relation to those with mental health problems and, thus, the potential of the policy for this population will not be realised. *A Vision for Change* highlights the cycle of exclusion for those with mental health problems. This cycle can lead to withdrawal from society, which in turn may lead to reduced quality of life, worsening mental health, loss of social networks, poverty and unemployment. Mental health problems are often episodic and prone to recur resulting in loss of income, loss of employment and consequently poverty. In addition, the developments of social contacts at work and in the community are often hampered.

2.5.1 Stigma and discrimination

Stigma and discrimination associated with mental ill health is pervasive and more than forty

negative consequences of stigma have been identified (Byrne, 1997). These include discrimination in housing, employment and education. Furthermore, it can lead to incidences of harassment for those living in the community. A study by MIND found that 50% of respondents with mental health problems had experienced harassment in the community and workplace (Read & Baker, 1996). A more recent study by Berzins *et al* (2003) found that people with mental health difficulties were twice as likely to experience harassment as people in the general population. Many of the fears and prejudices of the general public are based on myths about ill health (Social Exclusion Unit, 2004; Commission of European Communities, 2005). Individuals can experience stigma and discrimination even after symptoms have subsided (Social Exclusion Unit, 2004). In an Australian study, service users and their families identified 'less stigma' as the most important thing that would improve their lives (cited in Hocking, 2003), suggesting that stigma can act as a barrier towards optimal recovery. Furthermore, they reported that it was not just stigma from the community that affected their lives, but also stigma from healthcare workers. Education programmes aimed at tackling stigma and discrimination have shown positive results (Wolff *et al.,* 1996). The National Institute for Mental Health in England (NIMHF, 2004) published a five-year strategy aimed at tackling stigma and discrimination. The strategy is based on international evidence and is targeted at young people, media, health and social care providers, public and private organisations and the voluntary sector. Mental Health Ireland has run a debating competition to increase awareness of mental health problems in secondary schools. In addition, Schizophrenia Ireland (2005) launched a media-watch campaign to challenge the way schizophrenia is portrayed in the media. New Zealand campaigns aimed at tackling stigma have included the Like Minds project. Increased contact between the community and those with mental health difficulties has been shown to reduce the prejudice and stigma associated with mental illness (Couture & Penn, 2003). *A Vision for Change* recommended that issues of stigma and discrimination be addressed by developing and putting into action evidence-based programmes for the wider community.

2.5.2 Social isolation, community integration and participation

People with mental health problems report high levels of social isolation (MIND, 2004) and this is especially so for those with severe and persistent mental illness. Individuals in community residential facilities tend to have smaller social networks and these networks tend to be dominated by staff, professionals and other residents as opposed to friends from outside the services (Goering *et al*, 1992). The social networks of those with severe mental illness are significantly smaller than those of age-matched community controls (Becker *et al*, 1997). In addition, those with mental illnesses who have smaller networks tend to have more hospitalisations and make less use of external services (Becker *et al.*, 1997). Social networks improve for those who participate in programmes directly aimed at targeting social networks (Thornicroft & Breakey, 1991).

In terms of social integration, those relocated to community facilities tend to show an increase in contact with non-mental health services and engage in more leisure and social activities in the community (Shepherd & Murray, 2001).

However, the advantages of social integration may depend on the quality of the interactions as opposed to the quantity. An Italian study found that the number of activities offered in community residential facilities did not correlate with the residents' clinical and social functioning (de Girolamo *et al.*, 2002). It has been reported that community integration can be increased by moving activities (e.g. leisure, art) normally provided in mental health day facilities into the community and by providing activities in which the wider community can partake (Shepherd & Murray, 2001).

The Values to Action programme highlighted in *A Vision for Change* was specifically designed to address poor self-image, one of the factors that may prevent people from integrating and participating in the community. This programme was offered to mental health service users and staff. The staff felt that it enriched their role as mental health professionals and positive effects for the service users were also illustrated.

2.5.3 Employment

Those with mental health problems often find it difficult to secure or retain competitive employment. Competitive employment refers to a regular job, supervised by the employer, for regular wages and in an integrated work setting (Drake *et al*, 1999). The reported US rates for competitive employment of those with mental illness are low, and are typically less than 15% (cited in Drake *et al.*, 1999). In the UK, an employment rate of 24% for those with long term mental health problems has been reported (Rankin, 2005b). Yet research shows that a large proportion, between 60% and 70% of those with severe mental illness want to work in mainstream employment (Rankin, 2005). The barriers to employment include low self-esteem, low expectations of service users by staff, employer attitudes and difficulties moving from benefits to work (Social Exclusion Unit, 2004).

There is now a variety of services to meet the vocational and occupational needs of those with mental health problems. These range from day centres to supported employment programmes. Historically, sheltered workshops and day centres were provided by mental health services as an alternative to competitive employment. Sheltered work programmes include manual non-skilled work and skilled work such as carpentry, while day centres cater for the social care of the individual and may also provide vocational training. These workshops are based on the premise that those with severe mental illness are unsuited to competitive employment where the stress of the workplace would have detrimental effects on their mental health. Most often, individuals tend to become trapped in sheltered work programmes and the transition to competitive employment is never achieved (Drake *et al*, 1999). The pre-vocational workshops or 'train and place' programmes are provided in the mental health centre or similar setting and are aimed at providing the individual with the necessary skills for the real workplace. It is assumed that through these workshops the individual will gain the necessary skills for competitive employment in the real world. These programmes train the user on the assumption that the skills are transferable to the real workplace, with the goal of finding placement in competitive employment. However, the success of the transfer of skills from artificial environments to real-world settings is still being debated. Two types of open work programmes that are implemented in real-world settings and come under the 'place and train' model of employment, are the social co-

operatives and transitional employment. Social co-operatives are non-profit-making organisations that provide a valuable service to the community and employ an integrated workforce. The workforce is paid by the social co-operatives and the organisations receive a subsidy for each worker. The transitional employment model provides mental health service users with part-time and time-limited placements in the community. The service users are paid the prevailing wage, directly from the employer. The purpose of these programmes is to aid transition to competitive employment, develop the curriculum vitae and improve self-esteem. Very little scientific evidence for the success of these models exists (Thornicroft & Tansella, 2003). However, a study by Corrigan and McCracken (2005) showed that a place and train model increased the ability of people to attain their employment and housing goals compared with the traditional model of train and place.

More recently the supported employment model, as opposed to the traditional sheltered employment model, has become the preferred model of employment for those with severe mental illness. Research findings showed that supported employment models resulted in higher levels of competitive employment and higher earnings and that these positive effects increased over a 24-month period (Cook *et al.*, 2005). The supported employment model of 'place and train' proposes that individuals be placed in competitive employment and trained in the necessary skills. It emphasises a client-centred approach with employment specialists working closely with case managers and clinical teams. The team approach provides practical assistance in finding and maintaining employment. *A Vision for Change* highlighted the importance of the 'place and train' model. Another approach within the supported employment model is the 'choose, get and keep' approach (Bond et al., 1997). This approach emphasises career planning and choice of clients. As the name suggests, the approach helps clients to set goals, job search, choose suitable employment and secure placements. Ongoing support in terms of skill development and interventions when necessary is provided. Supported employment for people with severe mental illness is an evidence-based practice with resulting benefits for the individual's clinical and social functioning (Bond, 2004). The benefits of supported employment include improved self-esteem and better symptom control. It has recently been recommended that mental health services should include a variety of vocational training and employment options depending on user needs and aspirations. These options include approaches from both the sheltered employment model and the supported employment model (Thornicroft & Tansella, 2003). It is argued that choice and variety are important factors and that some form of meaningful activity is beneficial to the client's wellbeing, be that paid employment, voluntary employment or education and skills development (Rankin & Regan, 2004).

2.6 HOUSING MODELS OF RESIDENTIAL CARE

Johnson (2005) argued that quality housing is of paramount importance in community care and that safe and secure housing is one of the key factors for better quality of life and a 'place' within the local community. Shepherd and Murray (2001) argued that an adequate range of residential accommodation is at the core of attempts to develop community-based systems of care. The policy of bed reduction in hospitals in Ireland was accompanied by an increase in the responsibility of the mental health services for the management and provision of alternative accommodation for those in need. Two main models of housing are provided for those with severe mental illnesses – the sheltered housing model and the supported housing model.

2.6.1 Sheltered housing model

During the 1980s the prevailing model for community care was the continuum model, otherwise known as the sheltered housing model (Carling, 1993). Adherents of this model proposed that a variety of residential facilities should be created to provide a linear continuum of care from high to low levels of restrictiveness (Drachman, 1981; Wing & Furlong, 1986). This continuum model of care assumed that residents would move from high support to low support, with the final outcome being independent living in the community. Within this model the range of residential accommodation proved difficult to categorise. However in a UK study, Lelliott et al, (1996) proposed categories depending on level of staff cover, number of beds and staff to resident ratio. Four categories of community residential facilities, ranging from high support hostels to group homes were proposed. The majority of sheltered residential facilities now use these categories, or a version of them. The categories include:

- □ High support residences have nursing staff present 24 hours a day, with staff remaining awake at night-time;

- □ Medium support residences are staffed 24 hours a day, with staff sleeping at night-time;

- □ Low support residences are not staffed, but on-call staff are available when necessary. Staff visit on a regular basis during the day;

☐ Group homes are the least restrictive and are not staffed, although staff visit regularly.

The category of medium support residences in Ireland differs from that described above. Some medium support residences are not staffed throughout the day or at night, but have staff visiting daily. Other medium support residences have supervision at night by non-nursing staff. The low support residences and group homes have staff visiting occasionally. The lack of a standardised definition of support levels in Ireland has been a cause of concern. Definitions of levels of support adopted by this study were those put forward by the consultants of the specialised rehabilitation and recovery mental health teams and are detailed in Chapter 3.

The sheltered housing model of residential care has been strongly criticised by Carling (1993). He argued that the model confuses housing and treatment needs. Furthermore, alternative housing is often not available at the precise time that the person's need changes and frequent relocation can often upset or disrupt aftercare and social networks. The findings of studies investigating mobility between residential facilities do not support the sheltered housing model. An Italian study found very little mobility between residential facilities (de Girolamo et al., 2002) and results from a UK study indicated that residential facilities will probably be 'homes for life' for the majority of residents (Trieman et al., 1998). Likewise, Geller and Fisher (1993) in the US argued that the continuum model of residential care was never actualised and failed to function in the way in which it was intended. They found that only 7.9% of people were in residential placement that was less restrictive than their placement four years previously. Of the residents who

were judged as potentially suitable for independent living, only 16% were living independently at follow-up four years later.

Noteworthy is the comment made in the *Report of the Inspectorate of Mental Hospitals* (Department of Health and Children, 2004) regarding dependency and lack of mobility within the community residences:

> "The Inspectorate had been struck by how little rehabilitation took place in the community residences and how their management was oriented towards continuing care, rather than decreasing dependency. "

The report went on to add that the residences were over-staffed, did not have the proper skill mix of staff and that there was little investment in occupational rehabilitation or training for the residents.

2.6.2 Supported housing model

The supported housing model has replaced the notion of transitional care inherent in the sheltered housing model. This model emphasised permanent and supervised housing arrangements and has been widely accepted in the US and UK (Trieman et al, 1998). Advocates of the supported model proposed that independent living facilities be made available and services recently termed 'floating supports' be provided depending on the individual's level of need (Johnson, 2005; Rog, 2004). An important feature of the supported housing model is that return to independent living is not considered the ultimate goal. It is acknowledged that some residents will not return to independent living and that the provision of a flexible system of support allows for a fluctuating level of need. Thus, the objective of the intervention differs from that of the sheltered housing model of return to independent living. The Supporting People Programme in the UK recognises the importance of the supported housing model and of identifying local service need and co-ordinating funding for all supported housing services.

In summary, the sheltered housing model requires residents to move to a house to avail of different levels of support according to changing needs, while the supported housing model advocates permanency of housing for residents and a flexible support service that can be availed of when necessary to meet changing needs. In both models, a problem may arise if support is not matched to need. If needs are overprovided for, this may have negative consequences for the individual's functioning. It is suggested that, rather than having one model of care, both models could be incorporated in a service to suit the needs of individuals (Geller & Fisher, 1993; Johnson, 2005). For example, transitional housing may be beneficial to those who have been in long-term care and who require various levels of rehabilitation before moving to independent living. Supported housing may be more suitable to people who have not been hospitalised for long periods of time, but who may need a flexible level of care. Research investigating the effectiveness of supported housing versus other housing approaches has been scarce and equivocal (Shepherd & Murray, 2001; Rog, 2004). It would appear that housing with supports in any form increases housing stability, decreases homelessness and decreases hospitalisation (Rog, 2004). In addition, health care costs are reduced for those in higher-quality housing and neighbourhoods (Harkness et al., 2004). Furthermore, research suggests that the density of houses for socially marginalised groups, such as those with mental health problems, can affect re-hospitalisation rates and reduce

demand for mental health service interventions (Johnson, 2005). Too many houses in the same area may create a ghetto, while too few can lead to isolation and social exclusion.

2.7 PROVISION OF HOUSING AND CARE

Aside from the housing model adopted, the responsibility for the provision of housing within the mental health services has been an issue of debate for a number of years. The most common practice in Ireland has been that mental health services provide both housing and care. During the deinstitutionalisation programme, the mental health services provided housing for those being relocated from psychiatric hospitals. This housing was also used and continues to be used for those who come into contact with the mental health services and who cannot live without some form of support. *A Vision for Change* argued that local authorities should provide housing for service users in need, which is their obligation under the Housing Act 2002. However, the provision of housing by the mental health services has unfortunately resulted in reducing the chances of local authority housing for these individuals. In Sweden (Brunt & Hansson, 2004), housing for those with mental illnesses is provided by local authorities, while care is provided by health services. However, the UK provides an alternative model of independent sector providers.

2.7.1 Social housing in Ireland

The history of social housing in Ireland dates back to the Housing of the Working Classes Act of 1890. This legislation put in place mechanisms for allowing, if not obliging, local authorities to provide housing in urban areas. However, little progress was made until the Housing Act of 1919, was introduced which obliged local authorities to provide housing where it was needed, with the added incentive that subsidisation became available from central sources.

During the 1930s, large scale provision of urban housing for working people saw the establishment of housing estates where occupiers became tenants of the local authority on a rental basis. People were placed on a housing list in the growing local authority provision. This was the genesis of the waiting list phenomenon which persists to this day and which relied heavily on a points system in determining priority for families on the list, with points being allocated on the basis of number of children, health and other considerations. Progress slowed during the war of 1939 – 45 but accelerated in the 1950s and 1960s, and the legislative framework within which local authorities operated was extended and modernised by the Housing Act of 1966.

Possibly because the existing arrangements were perceived as encouraging dependence and inhibiting self-determination and because of financial considerations, two main considerations entered thinking in relation to local authority provision and central funding. The first was the encouragement of voluntary involvement, partly on a public/private basis, and the second the encouraging of tenants to become purchasers and owners of rented property. This new thinking was ratified in policy documents such as *A Plan for Social Housing* of 1991 and *Social Housing – the Way Ahead* of 1995. This latter publication aspired to an annual social housing provision of 7,000 new homes. The limiting factor in this aspiration was the rising price of land acquisition, the hoarding of land banks and increasing construction costs. In face of these considerations and problems, a series of further reports issued, collectively called *The Bacon Reports*, the last of which, *Action on Housing*, appeared in 2000. The

National Development Plan 2000 – 2006 included housing as an important element and allocated four billion Euro for social and affordable housing with the ambition, inter alia, of commencing 23,000 new social housing units in the local authority, voluntary and co-operative housing sectors over the three years 2006 to 2008. The Planning and Development Act of 2000, inter alia, empowered planning authorities to set aside 20% of housing developments for social and affordable housing and obliged local authorities to devise and implement housing strategies. Finally, the Department of the Environment published in 2005 a document titled *Housing Policy Framework – Building Sustainable Communities* in which there was an acknowledgement of the special housing needs of several groups, including persons with disabilities, encompassing persons with mental health disabilities, although this group was not specifically mentioned.

The central body charged with responsibility for housing issues is the Department of the Environment, Heritage and Local Government. The Department has a number of sections which impact on groups such as the elderly, travellers, etc, including the Housing Policy Section and the Social Inclusion Section, both based in headquarters in Dublin and the Voluntary Housing Section located in Ballina. The Government's *Homelessness: An Integrated Strategy* obliges local authorities to draw up action plans to provide a coherent response to homelessness. The Department assists local authorities to provide housing through its Capital Assistance Scheme, but the management and the maintenance of local authority housing is the authorities' own responsibility. The Capital Assistance Scheme has been something of an ad hoc arrangement and needs establishment on a continuing basis to remove uncertainty from the funding it provides.

While officially there are currently 45,000 – 50,000 persons awaiting local authority housing, there is scepticism in some quarters about the validity of this figure and a belief that the real number is substantially lower. It was reported that those persons who constitute family groupings can, at least in the Dublin area, be housed almost immediately although not necessarily in their location of choice. In contrast a study investigating social housing needs in a peripheral rural area argued that local authority housing lists grossly underestimate the housing need (Heaune, 2006). The author reported that people for a variety of reasons do not apply for local authority housing, especially those requiring special needs or sheltered social housing. To add to this, families are given priority in the allocation of local authority housing. Housing single persons who do not, in the ordinary sense, comprise a household, poses more difficulties, although authorities are embarking on providing apartments rather than the conventional three-bed roomed house hitherto regarded as the norm. In addition, some housing authorities consider persons in mental health community residences as housed and therefore not in need of housing, despite the fact that a small, but unknown, proportion of residents, particularly in group homes, are already on the housing waiting list. Additionally, local authorities view persons with psychiatric histories as potentially troublesome and feel that, even if they were to provide for them, they would get inadequate support from the mental health services in caring for their mental health needs. As recommended in *A Vision for Change* there needs to be close liaison between local housing authorities and mental health services to ensure that those who

need housing are housed and that sufficient care and support is provided to ensure wellbeing and successful tenancy.

It has been the rule that group homes have housed three to four persons and there is no reason why this grouping should not constitute a household for local authority housing purposes to avoid the obvious hazards of placing a person with mental health problems in the isolation of a single-occupancy apartment. Recently, novel schemes involving housing authorities entering into arrangements with landlords to provide tenancy sustainment services where the interest of the tenant are progressed and supported by the local administration are being developed.

In its preventative strategy targeted at specific groups the Homeless Agency includes 'people leaving mental health residential facilities' and sets out that all psychiatric hospitals will provide a formal and written discharge policy to service users and carers. Psychiatric teams will have a nominated professional acting as discharge officer and records will be kept of patients discharged and the accommodation to which they are being discharged. As distinct from prevention as envisaged above, there is no reference to the housing authorities' responsibility to provide for the housing requirements of those being discharged. In effect, it might be conceived that the document bars the discharge of patients who are homeless and requires the hospital or the mental health services to act as housing agents. In relation to providing for the mentally ill homeless in Dublin a number of specialist teams have been established. *A Vision for Change* recommended two full-time multidisciplinary teams for the Dublin area.

In no housing policy document is there a specific provision for the housing of persons with mental health problems and consequently the majority of the housing for those with mental illness in need of housing is provided by the mental health services. The mental health services provide most housing either on an owned or rented basis. However, a small housing stock, usually of three- to four-bedroom houses, for group home purposes is provided by some local housing authorities. In addition, a number of projects have been undertaken and realised by voluntary housing agencies, with some forming local housing associations, mostly with substantial grant aid from the Department of the Environment, Heritage and Local Government.

2.7.2 Housing provision for the mentally ill in the UK: an alternative model

In the UK, the National Health Service (NHS) and Community Care Act enabled agencies other than the NHS and local authorities to become involved in operating and managing residential facilities. This resulted in a greater involvement of non-statutory agencies (Shepherd & Murray, 2001). A large amount of affordable housing for those with mental health problems is provided by Registered Social Landlords. These may be industrial and provident societies, registered charities or companies. There are a number of different management and care arrangements for this type of housing. Firstly, the social landlords may hand over management responsibilities to voluntary organisations who take responsibility both for the housing management and care services. Secondly, the social landlord may take control of the housing management while entering into a support agreement with a care agency to provide care services. Alternatively, what is becoming

more common, the social landlord provides housing management and care services without the involvement of external agencies. Given the vast range of management and care providers, the National Housing Federation and the Mental Health Foundation (NHF/MHF) have produced a housing, care and support code (1996). The code lists 12 standards that organisations should commit to in order to achieve reliability and good quality in the care they provide. The Sainsbury Centre for Mental Health (Warner et al., 1997) produced a report on good practice in the provision of housing and support for people with mental health problems. This report covers all aspects of good practice, from the rights of the residents, staff training, individual care plans and the physical environment to the evaluation and monitoring of these supported housing arrangements.

In 2005, the Office of the Deputy Prime Minister (ODPM) published a guide to accommodation and support options for people with mental health problems. This guide discussed the support needs of people with mental health problems, the services provided by the Supporting People Programme and the range of housing and support options that are available. The purpose of this guide was to ensure that decision makers and health service providers were aware of and had access to important information on the range of services and options available to meet the needs of the service user.

Research on the evaluation of this type of provision (i.e. interagency working) has been limited and results have been equivocal. One of the first problems identified was that these services tended to take the 'easier' clients, leaving it more difficult to place those thought to be more 'difficult' (i.e. those with co-morbid problems, those who had contacts with police, those who had difficulties engaging with services) (Shepherd & Murray, 2001). Effective partnerships between statutory and non-statutory agencies required close interagency development. However as Shepherd and Murray (2001) point out, interventions for achieving effective partnerships have received little attention. The selection, recruitment and training of staff and management also have received little attention in terms of evaluative research. Finally, the expectations of residents and their preferences in terms of care have received little consideration. The NHF/MHF housing care and support code addresses all these issues. The code, however, was intended as a voluntary guide for those providing housing and care and to reward those organisations that met the standards. The Sainsbury report (Warner *et al.*, 1997) provides good practice guidelines on how to achieve these standards.

2.8 STAFF TRAINING IN RESIDENTIAL CARE

Studies have shown that a large proportion of the staff in community residential facilities have no formal training in mental health (de Girolamo & Bassi, 2004; Lelliott *et al.*, 1996). One UK survey reported that over half of the staff had no training, not even in risk or violence management (Lelliott *et al.*, 1996). This may be advantageous in that 'institutional attitudes' are not present. However, if the staff are not trained to deal with difficult situations, a residential facility may have to impose stricter selection criteria, resulting in difficult-to-manage individuals being refused admittance. The PRISM Psychosis Study (Thornicroft *et al.*, 1998) carried out in the UK argued that the quantity of the staff was not as important as the quality of the staff. It is more important to have the proper skill mix of staff, including psychiatrists, psychologists, nursing staff and care staff (Department of Health and

Children, 2006). In addition, all staff within residential facilities, regardless of profession or grade and including qualified and non-qualified staff, should be trained in the competencies and principles of recovery (MHC, 2005b). A document published by the New Zealand Mental Health Commission (2001) outlined the competencies necessary for mental health care workers and the Mental Health Commission in Ireland stressed that this is an invaluable document for services that are moving towards a recovery-based service.

As already mentioned, effective interagency co-operation is necessary to provide a comprehensive and seamless service. This should include health and social workers, housing agencies, occupational providers, primary care teams and police and probation officers. It should be borne in mind that the great majority of staff in Irish community residences, whether based therein or calling in on a daily basis, are trained psychiatric nurses who nevertheless require more specialised training in rehabilitation skills and in the competencies and principles of recovery.

2.9 RESIDENTIAL CARE IN THE COMMUNITY: A RESEARCH OUTLINE

Three main studies of the provision, range and adequacy of community mental health care facilities have influenced the methodology and procedures of the present study. Two of these were carried out in the UK (Lelliott *et al.*, 1996; O' Driscoll & Leff, 1993; Donnelly et al., 1994) and one in Italy (de Girolamo *et al.*, 2002). Both the UK studies surveyed a sample of residential facilities, while the Italian study surveyed community residential facilities throughout Italy.

In the UK, the Team for the Assessment of Psychiatric Services (TAPS) was established in 1985 to oversee and evaluate the move from hospital care to community care (O' Driscoll and Leff, 1993). This longitudinal study investigated the transition from hospital to community care over a five-year period. The findings regarding progression from high support hostels to low support and eventually to independent living showed very little mobility between differing levels of care, with 61% of the former patients remaining in the original placements. The authors proposed that, at least for patients who were resettled from hospital care, these hostels remained 'homes for life' for many (Trieman *et al*, 1998). Findings in relation to clinical and social outcomes were more positive (Leff & Trieman, 2000). While there was no change in the patients' clinical state or in problems of social behaviour, the residents had gained domestic and community living skills. A high percentage (84%) reported satisfaction with their current community accommodation and wished to remain there. Increases in social networks and more intimate relationships in the community were evident over the five-year period. Physical health declined for some residents, which was attributable to the age profile of the study group. This study was valuable in that it included measures directly aimed at the residents' views of their lives including accommodation and treatment. Regarding staff, in line with the findings of Lelliott *et al*, (1996), this study revealed that the majority of care staff had no formal qualifications. Training needs were not being met and there were few career opportunities (Senn *et al.*, (1997). Staff reported that while formal training was offered, it was often impossible to avail of due to limited budgets and workloads. This large-scale study highlighted the benefits of community care for long-stay patients resettled from large psychiatric hospitals.

A similar study was carried out in Northern Ireland – *Opening new doors* - to evaluate the move to community care (Donnelly et al., 1994). Interestingly, this study found that the majority of the patients went to staffed accommodation even though they had quite high skill levels. The skills level of the residents did not change over a two-year period and very few had moderate or major difficulties with daily living skills after six years (Donnelly *at al.*, 1997). In addition residents' views indicated that they preferred the community

accommodation over hospital and were more satisfied with their lives, felt healthier and felt more independent (Donnelly *et al.*, 1996). Regarding social support networks, a large proportion reported that they had no friends outside of the residence, twelve months following discharge, suggesting that residents were not easily integrating into the local community. The utilization of services 6 – 12 months following relocation showed that general practice, community psychiatric nurses and social workers were the mostly used services. Approximately a quarter were attending day centres and clubs, while only a small minority had gained open employment or sheltered employment (Mc Gilloway and Donnelly, 1998).

The Mental Health Residential Care Study by Lelliott *et al.*, (1996) assessed the provision of residential facilities within community mental health services in the UK. This study employed a facility questionnaire and resident questionnaire. The facility questionnaire was gathered by interviewing service managers, while the resident questionnaire provided information for each resident from the individual's key worker. In terms of community residential facilities, the main finding was the categorisation of facilities into high, medium and low support, based primarily on the staff to resident ratio and the extent of cover. There was wide variation in the training of staff, with more than half of the staff having no formal qualifications. There was very little support from external services, such as visits from psychiatrists, psychologists, social workers or community psychiatric nurses. The majority of residents had long-term mental illness, with over 62% having had a first contact with mental health services more than 10 years previously. The majority were diagnosed as having schizophrenia. A large number (56%) had a physical disability or had had physical health problems in the last month. Those in the high support hostels were the most vulnerable and most impaired in activities of daily living when compared with resident groups in medium and low staffed hostels, acute wards and group homes. The study identified those receiving residential care in the 1990s and made some attempt at classifying residences according to extent of care and staff to resident ratio. However, the study did not address the physical environment of the residences, the management polices or the rehabilitative efforts of the different levels of facility to integrate the residents into the community. While the study did include a residents' profile, this was completed by the staff and not by the residents themselves. This imposes a number of limitations. Firstly, the majority of staff were untrained, bringing into question the validity of their subjective judgements of the residents' levels of functioning and diagnoses. Secondly, no attempt was made to ascertain the residents' satisfaction with the facilities and services. And finally, no effort was made to quantify the subjective quality of life of the residents.

The Italian study (de Girolamo et al., 2002; de Girolamo & Bassi, 2004) was a national survey of non-hospital residential facilities in Italy. It included measures from both TAPS (O' Driscoll & Leff, 1993) and the British Residential Care Study (Lelliott et al., 1996). This was a two-phase study with the first phase surveying all facilities based in the community with four or more residential places. The first phase was a census of all the aforementioned facilities and looked at the provision of services, staffing, and patient demographics. Results were very much in line with those of previous work in the UK (Lelliott et al., 1996; Trieman et al., 1998) and the US (Geller & Fisher, 1993) in that there was very little mobility between the residences, approximately 40% of staff had no formal qualifications and the majority of the residents were diagnosed with schizophrenia. The residents differed from those in the UK studies in that the majority (48%) had never been admitted to inpatient care, although the median length of illness was 22 years. In the UK studies, the residents had all been relocated from psychiatric hospitals. The second phase involved a random sample of 20% of all residences. It included two schedules – the structure schedule and the patient schedule. The structure schedule covered all aspects of the facilities from

organisation, treatment plans, staffing, external and internal rehabilitative activities to linkages to other facilities. The findings suggest that the physical environment, the size and the staffing pattern in terms of quantity and skill mix of staff may have influenced the residents' quality of life and created a more home-like environment (Picardi et al., 2006). The patient schedule included items such as diagnosis, pattern of symptoms, appropriateness of placement, former place of residence and prediction of place of residence in six months. This schedule also included the Health of the Nation Outcome Scale (HoNOS), the Global Assessment of Functioning (GAF) and the Physical Health Index (PHI). Few managers judged residents as having short-term prospects of discharge and discharge to independent living was uncommon (Santone et al., 2005). The majority of the residences had one or more type of rehabilitative activity either internal or external to the facility, with only 12% providing no rehabilitative activity. Interestingly, there was no association between the intensity of the rehabilitative activities (i.e. the number of activities provided) and the staff ratings of the residents' functioning. The authors suggested that quality may have been a more important factor than quantity. This large-scale study provided important information on the provision and type of residential care in Italy. It extended the work previously carried out in the UK by including process of care items such as the provision of internal and external rehabilitation facilities. However, one of the limitations of the study was the failure to obtain the residents' views.

A review of the literature revealed that the majority of users would prefer independent living arrangements with flexible staff levels (Shepherd, 1998). It is argued that common indicators of quality of care in residential facilities include the quality of the physical environment, individualisation of care, privacy, autonomy and the attractiveness of the neighbourhood. These quality of care factors have been shown to be related to quality of life measures (Shepherd & Murray, 2001) such as satisfaction with treatment and care, food, accommodation and relationships with others. Furthermore, the differences in quality of life ratings between community-based residents and hospital-based patients seemed to be the result of apparently minor factors such as access to kitchens, choice at mealtimes, being able to lock the bathroom door and access to one's own television. The results would suggest that quality of care items such as these are indeed linked to subjective satisfaction and quality of life.

It must be kept in mind that independent living is not always feasible for some individuals often because of treatment-resistant psychotic illness (Macpherson & Jerrom, 1999). An appropriate alternative is the 24-hour nursing facility; individuals placed in these services have been shown to have improved social functioning and report higher satisfaction than those in institutions (Shepherd, 1998). The increase in functioning resulted in approximately 40% of those referred being able to move to less supervised settings within two to three years (Shepherd, 1998). However, this option still remains unattractive to many service users, specially the younger patients who demand a certain level of autonomy and privacy, but may require high levels of support with management of money, preparation of food and other social amenities. Thus, a 24-hour service must ensure that it meets the needs of these service users so that it is an accepted service that encourages and promotes recovery. The balance between users' preferences and a cost-effective and safe level of care will not be achieved without the combination of community-based housing with support from highly specialised rehabilitation and recovery mental health teams who adhere to a recovery ideology.

2.10 THE PRESENT STUDY

The Mental Health Research Division (MHRD) of the Health Research Board (HRB) has over the years carried out health service research in the mental health area. The first study in the series was a review of the availability and utilisation of acute psychiatric beds (Keogh et al., 1999). The second was a review of the purposes and functions of day hospitals and day centres (Hickey et al., 2003). The third in the series – the present study – reviews the provision, functions and purposes of residential services. Significant changes to mental health policy, coupled with the lack of previous mental health services research into community residential care, led to the funding of this important study by the Mental Health Commission and the Health Research Board.

The study aimed to describe and investigate the function of community residences with reference to the appropriateness of the premises and the extent to which the residence meets the needs of the residents. Residents themselves were the prime reporters as to their views of their lives and their levels of satisfaction with current service provision. The interaction of residents with the community and their satisfaction with their neighbourhood and environment was also investigated. Enquiry was made as to their 'citizenisation', i.e. they were on the Register of Electors, whether they used communal social amenities, participated in local activities and used general health care services. In addition, staff perceptions of the aims and functions of the residences were investigated, as well as their perceptions of the factors that impeded or promoted independent living. It was envisaged that the study would make recommendations regarding the appropriate structures and functions of community residences and the necessary programmes, mechanisms and conditions to promote independent living, self-reliance and community integration. The specific aims of the study were to:

☐ Examine the physical environment of the residential facilities

☐ Report on the demographic and clinical profile of residents

☐ Examine the staffing, management and care practices in the facilities

☐ Investigate residents' levels of disability and of clinical, physical and social functioning and the extent to which impairments and disabilities reduced performance of everyday living activities

❑ Investigate residents' satisfaction with care and treatment, accommodation and other aspects of their lives

❑ Determine the extent to which civil rights were met

❑ Report on the perceived functions of the residences and the extent to which they met the residents' needs.

both service providers' perceptions and service users' views. Given the current climate of policy development and service change in Ireland, research of this kind is particularly necessary. The present study attempts to remedy a current deficit in this area.

2.11 SUMMARY

This chapter has defined what community care means for mental health service personnel and the problems associated with the move to community-based care. Models of housing provision for those with severe and persistent mental illness, together with considerations relevant to their effective operation, particularly in relation to rehabilitation, have been reviewed. There has been a change in recent years in Ireland, albeit gradual, to a recovery philosophy emphasising the principles of individual choice, partnership, empowerment and control. However, recent documents have highlighted the importance of the recovery-oriented services (Department of Health and Children, 2006; Mental Health Commission, 2005b). The move to community care in Ireland has been ongoing for over 30 years. The move has been unstructured and variable across the country. In addition, no evaluations on a national level of the community residential facilities or the treatment and care in these facilities have taken place. Local mental health service research has taken place; the importance of this research for local service planning and development cannot be over-emphasised. Of particular importance in terms of the recovery philosophy are the residents' perceptions of their lives and their satisfaction with services, and the level of autonomy within their lives.

It is important that research informs policy as to the best way forward in service planning and delivery, taking into account

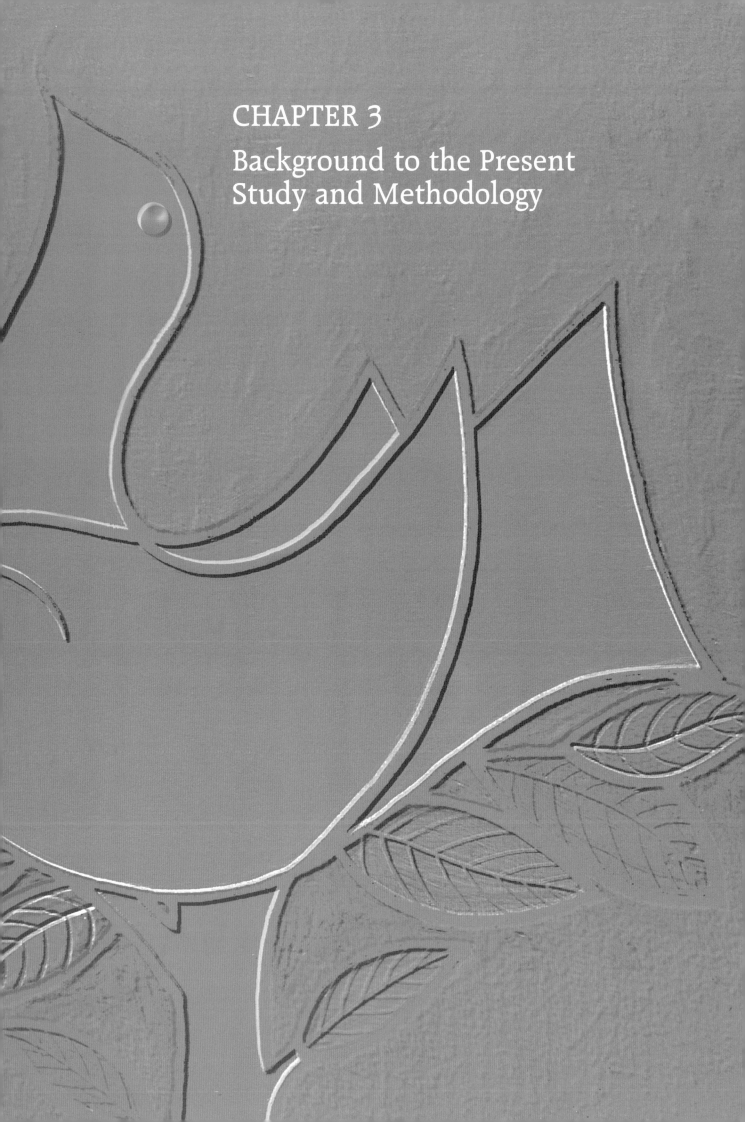

CHAPTER 3
Background to the Present Study and Methodology

Chapter 3

Background to the present study and methodology

3.1 INTRODUCTION

The current study was conducted during the period 01/06/04 to 31/05/06 and employed both qualitative and quantitative methods. Questionnaires were designed to evaluate the residential facilities, collect demographic information, assess the clinical and psychosocial functioning of the residents and perceptions of the residents and staff. Quantitative data were augmented by qualitative information gathered from open-ended questions, informal observation and social interactions in the course of fieldwork. During data collection, the primary researcher spent time in the residences observing and talking with the staff and residents.

A two-phase procedure was adopted in the study. The first phase of the study involved the completion of questionnaires by directors of nursing for all community residential facilities in the three HSE areas. The returned questionnaires were then used to classify the residences as high, medium or low support using the following definitions:

◻ High support - 24-hour nursing care

◻ Medium support – supervision (non-nursing) at night, with staff member visiting regularly

◻ Low support – no supervision at night, with staff visiting regularly.

The next phase involved the random selection of a sample of high, medium and low support facilities within each catchment area in the three participating HSE areas. From these, a random sample of residents was selected to be interviewed.

In addition, staff present in the selected residences completed a questionnaire regarding the aim and function of community residences and the factors that promote or impede return to independent living.

3.2 STUDY AREAS

The study began in June 2004, prior to the restructuring of the health services (see Section 1.4). At the beginning of the study, the health service was structured by health board area. Three health board areas were selected for participation in the study, based on their geographical location (rural or urban), their provision of a representative range of residential accommodation and their willingness to participate. Following the restructuring of the health service, the three health board areas became three HSE local areas within two HSE administrative regions. However, as already mentioned (Section 1.4), few changes had occurred at the time of the study in the management and delivery of the mental health services despite the implementation of the new structures in 2005.

The three HSE local areas that participated in the study are outlined in Chapter 1. For reasons of confidentiality, they will be referred to as HSE local areas A, B and C. Within these three HSE local areas there were a total of eight catchment areas each representing individual services. Table 3.1 shows the population figures for the individual catchment areas and total population figures for the HSE local areas (MHC, 2005a). HSE area C had the largest population. The total populations for those over 16 years of age were 384,236 in area C, 262,249 in area B and 168,867 in area A. The adult mental health services provided services for all those over 16 years of age in the population. In one catchment area in Area B – area B3 – community services were provided by this area but inpatient services were provided by another local area service, which was not participating in the study. However, there were no community residences in the B3 catchment area. While catchment area B3 is included in the population numbers for completeness, it is excluded from all other analyses.

Table 3.1   Population figures for study catchment areas and HSE local areas

CATCHMENT AREA	POPULATION*
Catchment A1	129, 008
Catchment A2	93, 754
Total Area A	*222, 762*
Catchment B1	175, 304
Catchment B2	103, 277
Catchment B3	61, 010
Total Area B	*339, 591*
Catchment C1	143, 029
Catchment C2	133, 559
Catchment C3	210, 346
Total Area C	*486, 934*

Source: Census 2002

Area A has the lowest population, is primarily rural and spans a wide geographical area. The physical geography of the area and the lack of public transport made it difficult to ensure that services were accessible to all. One of two catchment areas with community residences in Area B (Catchment B1) is primarily urban, while the other (Catchment B2) is primarily rural. Area C has also got one catchment area which is largely urban, while the remaining two are more rural. Area C includes some of the most deprived inner-city electoral areas. The tendency for a drift of disadvantaged persons to inner city areas, poor housing and the lack of social or family support resulted in a greater demand for mental health services in these areas. More information on the mental health services in the three study areas is provided at the end of this chapter in order to contextualise the study findings.

3.3   STUDY PARTICIPANTS

All community residential facilities (n = 102) in the three participating areas completed a questionnaire for the first phase of the study. The total number of returned questionnaires was validated with the liaison person within the area. Following this the facilities were classified into high, medium and low support. A stratified random sample (based on the level of support) of the residences from each of the catchment areas (see Section 3.2) were selected for participation in the next phase of the study. Based on the figures from the Report of the Inspector of Mental Hospitals (2003), it was envisaged that approximately 40% of the total residences would be included in the next phase of the study. A total of 43 residences were selected for participation in the next phase resulting in 42% (43 / 102) of the total number of residences.

For individual interview a random sample of residents was selected from the high, medium and low residences. The sample of residents from the different levels of support was in proportion to the total number of residents in each support setting. The target sample size was 120 residents and over-sampling was necessary to ensure that those who refused to participate could be replaced. Of all residents in the residences at the time of the study, approximately 16% (138 / 871) were interviewed. Similar proportions were interviewed from each of the three study areas (15% from local area A; 14% from local area B and 19% from local area C). Of those who were asked to participate in the study, sixteen (10%; 16 / 154) refused. The final sample interviewed resulted in a total of 15% (82 / 552) of the total high, 16% (25 / 153) of the total medium and 19% (31 / 164) of the total low support residents.

Staff questionnaires were only given to those residences that were selected for the second phase of the study. A total of 52 staff returned questionnaires. As actual numbers of staff were not recorded at the time of the study, the percentage of staff who returned the questionnaires is calculated from the return of staff numbers on the facility questionnaire. It is estimated that the 52 staff who returned questionnaires account for approximately 36% of total staff, including nursing staff and care staff. The estimated percentage of nursing staff returning questionnaires was 37% (39 / 105) and the estimated number of care staff returning questionnaires was 22% (9/40).

3.4 MEASURES

The study incorporated a total of four questionnaires – Facility Questionnaire, Residents Questionnaire, Key Worker Questionnaire and Staff Questionnaire (see Appendix 1 - 4). All the aims of the current study could not be met by any existing questionnaire, therefore in addition to standardised questionnaires, measures were developed and customised to meet the study aims. International research guided the questionnaire design. The Facility Questionnaire, Resident Questionnaire and Key Worker Questionnaire were informed by three international studies (de Girolamo et al., 2002; Lelliott, et al., 1996; Trieman et al., 1998). The Staff Questionnaire was designed primarily to gather information on the staff's perceptions of the aims of the residential facilities and factors that promoted or impeded return to independent living within the Irish context. The content and context validity of the questionnaires was ensured through

consultation with key stakeholders and relevant experts (i.e. Advisory Committee for the study, MHC, researchers, service providers, mental health managers and service users). A summary of the sections within each of the questionnaires are detailed in Table 3.2 and is followed by a brief description of each.

3.4.1 Facility questionnaire

This questionnaire was informed mainly by the study by de Girolamo et al (2002) and amended to suit to Irish context. The questionnaires were completed by the nursing officers in charge of the residence (see Section 3.5). There were a total of 13 sections in the questionnaire (Table 3.2). The following section summaries each section (See Appendix 1 for specific questions). For ease of reading, information on the scoring of the scales are also given in the appropriate place in the results sections.

- *Building features* - ownership of building, location, and number, type and use of rooms. *Access to services* - time to reach other frequently used services such as GP, shopping and post office.

- *Rules and regulations* – rules govern the residents daily activities, privacy and control over finances.

- *Meals* – who prepares the meals

- *Staff* – number of staff, shifts and emergency staff

- *Admission procedures* – formal admission procedures, exclusion criteria, bed use, ownership of beds and specialised rehabilitation teams.

- *Meetings* – type and frequency of meetings in the residence.

- *Evaluation process and procedures* – annual planning, evaluation of quality services and control, assessment of residents.

Table 3.2   Factors addressed in each of the four questionnaires

Facility questionnaire	Resident questionnaire	Key worker questionnaire for resident	Staff questionnaire
Building features	Demographic information	Psychiatric history	Aims / functions of residence
Access to services	Activities	Global Assessment of Functioning	
Rules / Regulations	Harassment		Factors that impede independent living
Food preparation	Satisfaction of treatment / care	Physical Health Index	
Wardrobe		Health of the Nation Outcome Scale	Factors that promote independent living
Staff	Quality of Life		
Admission procedures	Disability Assessment Scale	Disability Assessment Scale	
Meetings	Social Support		
Evaluation processes	BPRS		
Files/regulations	Perception of life in residence		

Resident characteristic
Activities
Community integration

☐ *System files and regulation* – health and safety, rights of residents, complaints and health initiatives.

☐ *Resident characteristics* - number, age, gender, diagnosis and employment.

☐ *Activity* – activities offered to residents e.g. social skills, employment type, physical activity, education and support activities.

☐ *Community integration* – activities that promote community integration such as integrated social activities and activities to facilitate re-housing and employment.

3.4.2 Resident questionnaire

The resident questionnaires were completed at the individual interviews with the sample of residents. See Table 3.2 for sections within the questionnaire and Appendix 2 for specific items within the sections. This questionnaire gathered information on demographic information, activities of the residents and if they had experienced harassment in the community. It also contained five questionnaires, detailed below.

☐ *Satisfaction with treatment and care* – this questionnaire was based on a section of the Core Assessment and Outcomes Packages for Mental Health Services (FACE Recording & Management Systems, 2000), which is widely used as an evaluation tool in the UK and NI and has recently been used by some services in Ireland (e.g. HSE Mid Western Area, HSE Northern Area). Only Your Treatment and Care questionnaire was used in the current study to assess the service users' experience of treatment and care. It contains a total of 22 items assessing the service users' knowledge of care plans and relationships with key workers and psychiatrists. Service users indicate their response to the statements by 'yes', 'no' or 'not sure'. Two general questions, using a four point scale, enquiring about the overall satisfaction of the residents with treatment and care and the information they received was assessed at the end of the questionnaire.

❏ *Quality of life* - the quality of life measure used was loosely based on the Satisfaction for Life Domains Scale (Tempier *et al.,* 1997) measuring satisfaction with life in general and in 17 life domains (see Appendix 2). Residents indicated their satisfaction on a three-point scale from 0 – 2, with higher scores indicating greater satisfaction. The scores on the 18 items were summed to give a total quality of life score.

❏ *Disability Assessment Scale (WHO DAS II)* – this scale measured functioning and disability in the last thirty days. It assessed functioning and disability in six domains including understanding and communication, getting around, self-care, getting along with others, household and work activities and participation in society. Both residents and the residents' key worker completed a version of this scale, resulting in two measures for each resident. The scale contains 12 items and is rated on a five-point scale from 0 – 4.

❏ *Social support* – the scale used to measure social support was similar to the Mannheim Interview on Social Support (Veiel, 1990) in that it asked about social support in four domains including everyday psychological support, everyday instrumental support, instrumental crisis support and psychological crisis support (see Section 6.1.1 for more details). Residents were asked to indicate who they asked for help during these times.

❏ *Brief Psychiatric Rating Scale (BPRS)* – this is a widely used measure within psychiatry and was employed to measure the resident's current psychopathology. The 24 symptoms were rated by the researcher on a seven-point scale (i.e. 1 = not present to 7 = extremely severe).

❏ *Perception of life in the residence* – this scale was devised by the authors to measure the residents' perceptions of live in the residence. Residents rated their perceptions on 12 areas including living in the house, how well residents got on together and with staff, how much control they had to lead their live as they wanted and how happy they were with their level of independence. At the end of the resident questionnaire, residents were asked an open-ended question regarding their life in the residence and what it was like to live there (see Section 8.5).

3.4.3 Key worker questionnaire for resident

The key worker questionnaire was employed to gather further information about the resident. It included psychiatric history, system of support, appropriateness of placement, general functioning, physical health, psychopathology and disabilities. See Appendix 3 for specific items on the questionnaire. Below is a short description of the standardised measures used.

☐ *Global Assessment of Functioning* (GAF American Psychiatric Association, 1994) – provides the clinician's judgement of the individual's overall level of functioning. The GAF scale is rated with respect to psychological, social and occupational functioning only and does not include impairment due to health or environmental limitations. The key worker rated the resident on a scale from one to 100.

☐ *Physical Health Index*– this is a simple measure for assessing physical health and has been used by the UK study (O'Driscoll and Leff, 1993) and the Italian study (di Girolamo *et al.*, 2005). This measured physical health problems on a scale of 0 – 3 with higher scores indicating greater disability. It is also used to rate the level of assistance required for disabilities on a scale of 0 – 7, again with higher scores indicating greater assistance required. Health in eight domains is assessed.

☐ *Health of the Nation Outcome Scale (HoNOS)* – this scale was designed to assess psychopathology and disability in the previous two-weeks and has previously been used in the Italian study (di Girolamo and Bassi, 2004). The scale measured clinical and social functioning in 11 domains using a five-point scale from 0 (no problems) to 4 (severe problems).

☐ *Disability Assessment Scale (WHO DAS II)* – key workers rated the residents on the DAS, as described above.

3.4.4 Staff questionnaire

The staff questionnaire was designed by the authors to assess the staff perceptions of the aims and functions of the residences and the factors that promoted or impeded return to independent living for the residents (see Appendix 4). Following the demographic information section, the staff were provided with a list of eight possible aims and functions of the residence and were asked to rate the importance of each on a scale from 1 (no importance) to 4 (greatest importance). They were then asked open-ended questions regarding the three main factors that they felt positively and negatively influenced return to independent living.

3.5 PROCEDURE

All research instruments were piloted before fieldwork proper began and adjustments were made to instruments and procedures as needed. Following experience gained from the pilot study, the following procedure was adopted during fieldwork. The researcher contacted the director of nursing regarding completion of the facility questionnaires. These were circulated by the director of nursing to the nursing officers in charge of the residences. The principle researcher's name and telephone number were included in all correspondence, ensuring that nurses had a contact number for any questions or queries that might arise. Completed questionnaires were returned to the director of nursing who returned them to the researcher. Following the return of the questionnaires the director of nursing identified a person with whom the researcher could liaise for the second phase of the study. The liaison person in the majority of instances was an assistant director of nursing.

A random sample of high, medium and low support residences was selected for the second phase of the study. The liaison person was informed of the residences selected, the approximate number of interviews required, the requirement of the key worker or staff nurse to complete a questionnaire for every resident interviewed, and suitable dates for interviewing. The contact person then informed the clinical nurse manager of the residences of the visit and the nurses informed the residents. The clinical nurse manager provided the researcher with a list of residents' names, excluding all those with organic brain injury and those in respite beds for less than three months. The interviews took place in the residential facilities or in some cases at a day care centre. The researcher arranged evening meetings for those residents that were not available during the day.

Prior to the interview, the researcher met with the resident and explained the content, context and purpose of the study. Conditions for study participation were explained to residents both verbally and summarised in a written summary of information given to participants before written consent was obtained. Participants were assured verbally and in writing that no personal identifying information would be recorded on the research instruments, that the information they disclosed would not be available to staff or other residents and would be used in the research report in a manner which would not allow for identification of the respondents. The information sheet explained that the information collected would be available to the research team only and that the questionnaires and other research materials would be destroyed in accordance with the HRB's record management policy (i.e one year following publication of study). Residents were informed that unwillingness to participate would not affect their treatment and care, and that they were free to take a break in the middle or withdraw from the interview at any time. They were also informed that a nurse would complete another questionnaire detailing their psychiatric history and clinical, social and occupational functioning. If the resident agreed to participate, they signed the study consent form and the interview began.

On completion of the interview with the resident, the key worker questionnaire was given to the key worker or nursing staff member. In most instances, there was no assigned key worker and the questionnaire was given to the nursing staff for completion. These questionnaires were completed on site in the majority of residences. However, in some instances, especially in the low and medium support facilities, there was no nurse on hand to complete the key worker questionnaire. In these instances the questionnaires were left with the liaison person to distribute to the appropriate nursing staff. These questionnaires were returned by post to the researcher when completed.

Nursing or care staff members who were on duty on the day of the visit completed the staff questionnaires. In addition, questionnaires were left at the site for completion by fellow staff members and were posted back to the researcher. All staff questionnaires were anonymous.

3.6   ETHICAL APPROVAL

International best practice (e.g. WHO, 1999) in relation to the conduct of ethical research in the social sciences informed the selection of methods and procedures for the present study. A Research Advisory Committee was established to advise on the project. The committee included representatives from the MHC, user groups and from the participating HSE areas.

The study proposal underwent internal and external peer review following the procedure set down by the HRB. The study received ethical approval from the HRB Research Ethics Committee (REC) in October 2004. Ethical approval for the study was also received from the REC in each of the catchment areas of the HSE areas. For those areas where there was no REC in place, approval was sought from the clinical directors. In addition, briefing meetings were held in each HSE area to inform service managers, staff and users about the study and to obtain their views.

3.7 DATA ANALYSIS

Analysis of the data was primarily descriptive. In most cases, descriptive statistics are presented , by level of support of the residence (i.e. high support, medium support and low support). Chi-square tests (with Yates' correction for 2 x 2 tables) were used to analyse categorical variables. The chi-square results are not reported when more than 20% of cells had an expected frequency of less than five. T-test or one-way analysis of variance (ANOVA) were used as appropriate to study differences in the mean of continuous variables between groups. ANOVA was followed by post-hoc comparisons according to the Bonferroni method. Non-parametric statistics were used to examine variables not normally distributed. As not all questions were answered on the questionnaires, degrees of freedom may differ throughout the report. SPSS Text Analysis for Surveys was used to analyse the qualitative data.

3.8 CONTEXTUALISING THE PARTICIPATING HSE LOCAL AREAS

In order to contextualise the results, it was necessary to provide some background information to the study areas. The information was obtained from clinical directors, directors of nursing and general managers of the services in the areas. Background documentation was gathered and unstructured interviews were carried out in the three HSE local areas. Information was gathered on the development and the characteristics of the mental health services and the context in which service developments occurred. Data included information on the philosophy and the aims of the residential facilities. In addition, the wider societal and environmental aspects of the study areas were investigated and their impact on mental health services and their users was explored. The role and function of related statutory and voluntary agencies in the areas were investigated. The following descriptions are based on the interviewer's notes of the meetings with service managers and providers.

3.8.1 *Resettlement of patients*

In HSE Area A, resettlement of patients into community residences in their local communities began in the mid-eighties. The philosophy underlying the community residential facilities, at least for the high support, supervised residential units (SRUs), was that these houses were 'homes for life' where treatment and care would be provided in a homelike environment. Properties were acquired on an ad hoc basis, with facilities selected on the basis of availability, size and affordability. Rehabilitation to prepare residents for the move was provided within the hospital by nursing staff prior to relocation. The staff played an important role in the continuing care of the residents in terms of monitoring medication and providing education and training in social skills and daily living skills. In Area A, the move to residential care in the community occurred over a relatively short period of time and was accompanied by the closure of one of the two large psychiatric hospitals in the area (in 1991). While the remaining hospital had been retained, it now has only two long-stay wards remained accommodating approximately 20 patients. It was reported that the lack of places in supervised residential facilities prevented the move of eight patients, while twelve patients were unsuitable for community care and needed to be accommodated elsewhere. A regional special care unit in the area accommodated eight patients. It was anticipated that the function of this unit would be readdressed in the near future, and attempts would be made to find more suitable accommodation for its clients.

The resettlement of patients to community residential care in Area B was similar to that in Area A and began in the mid-eighties following the publication of *Planning for the Future* in 1984. The underlying ethos here again was that the facilities were 'homes for life', with the staff helping the residents to adjust to life in the community. Basic assessments took place in a 'filter' ward in the hospital. The nurses had the responsibility of selecting those whom they deemed suitable for relocation to the community. The initial houses were medium or low support (they did not have 24-hour nursing care), but some of these were later redefined as high support. Attempts were made to get ordinary, large houses and to link the patients with the community from whence they came. The main criteria for the acquisition of premises were that they were in 'normal' type environments – neither deprived nor affluent areas – and were accessible to amenities such as churches, shops and bus services. One of the two large hospitals closed in Area B in 1999. The remaining hospital catered for 118 long-stay patients.

The resettlement in Area C began prior to *Planning for the Future* (1984). As early as the 1970s there were patients sleeping in community residential facilities in some areas in area C, but spending their days in the psychiatric hospital. This arrangement had evolved because of the large number of houses that were once provided for staff working in the hospital and were no longer required. For those services where resettlement had already begun, *Planning for the Future* recommended that emphasis should be placed on independent living through rehabilitation and re-socialisation programmes. For the services that did not have a resettlement programme already in place, *Planning for the Future* stressed that deinstitutionalisation and the process of rehabilitation and resettlement should begin. While the community residences were designed to provide step-down accommodation for those who on discharge from hospital could not live in their own homes, there was limited success in moving people on. As in the other areas, the process of deinstitutionalisation was regarded by many within the service, both staff and patients, as the provision of a 'home for life' for those relocated from the hospital. A study in Area C (Health Service Executive, 2004) reported that staff and professionals described the majority of residents as needing a 'home for life'. There were two large institutions in area C, which accommodated approximately 200 long-stay patients.

In summary, the resettlement of patients from large institutions and thus the development of community residences began in some areas in Ireland as early as 1960. In these areas resettlement was slow and only involved those who were least impaired. There were few or no rehabilitation or re-socialisation programmes in place. The resettlement of patients from large institutions gathered momentum in the 1980s with the publication of *Planning for the Future* (1984).

It was reported in all areas that, while government policy was behind the move, backing in terms of resources was meagre. Nurses and others within the hospitals undertook the rehabilitation and re-socialisation functions. Community accommodation was purchased where available and modified appropriately. Given the continued scarcity of resources, the development of community residential services was slow.

While all the three areas studied had begun the process of deinstitutionalisation, they were at different stages of evolution in this process at the time of the study. A number of service managers and providers pointed out that the philosophy of the community residential facilities at the time was that the patients were moving to their new homes, which would be homes for life. A large number of these residents still remained in the community residences to which they had come from inpatient care. For these residents, the community residential facilities have functioned as continuing care facilities.

3.8.2 Characteristics of the general mental health services in the three areas studied

Area A had a large number of psychiatric nurses in both catchment areas, with the majority employed in bed-based facilities. A large proportion of these nurses were attached to community residences. This left little resource for community-based care, and community mental health teams had been slow to develop. There was an insufficient number of multidisciplinary community health teams and a number of professionals worked in isolation, taking referrals from various sources, including direct referrals from primary care. There was a lack of resources for the development of multidisciplinary teams and there was a need for more professionals in clinical psychology, social work and occupational therapy. There were no specialist rehabilitation services; however, one catchment area was expected to have a specialist rehabilitation psychiatrist in post in the near future.

Both catchment areas in Area B had community mental health teams in operation although there was a shortfall in the number of teams. In addition, the teams were not adequately staffed with the necessary professionals, particularly in social work and occupational therapy. There was only one specialised rehabilitation team.

Community mental health teams were in operation in all catchment areas in Area C although there was a critical shortage of core staff. In one catchment there were no clinical psychologists or social workers. Catchment Area C2 had three management bodies, which included the HSE and two hospital boards in the area. There was only one specialised multidisciplinary rehabilitation team, and it was significantly understaffed.

3.8.3 Management of the mental health services

It was reported in the background interviews that the mental health services were managed on a regional level and on a catchment area level. The role of the regional management unit included funding, accountability and governance, planning, policy setting, and performance management. The regional management team also oversaw external relations with other bodies (HSE, MHC) and collaborations with other services, such as voluntary groups and local authorities. The catchment management teams' roles and responsibilities focused on the delivery of services and clinical leadership. The catchment management teams were consultant-led multidisciplinary teams. They had responsibility for local service provision and clinical leadership. In addition, there were consultant-led sector management teams that had an operational role within the sector. In some cases, members of the sector multidisciplinary team were shared with other sectors. As noted above, two of the catchment areas in the study had dedicated rehabilitation teams, yet neither of these teams had the full complement of multidisciplinary staff.

The referrals for the community residential facilities in all areas came exclusively from the sector teams. The responsibility for placement differed across the catchment areas. In four of the seven catchment areas, decisions about admissions and discharges to community residential care were the responsibility of the consultant-led teams. In two of the catchment areas, referrals were made to the dedicated rehabilitation psychiatrist and placement decisions were made in conjunction with the multidisciplinary rehabilitation team. In one of the catchment areas, placement was co-ordinated by a multidisciplinary rehabilitation placement committee. This committee was led by the assistant director of nursing.

3.8.4 Aims and functions of the community residential facilities

It was reported at the interviews with service managers, clinical directors and directors of nursing that the community residential facilities had become a continuing care facility for those relocated from the psychiatric hospitals. This was due mainly to the fact, that in the past, that both staff and residents believed that this indeed was the function of the residences. There was very little in the way of formal rehabilitation except for that offered by nursing staff. Residents helped about the house with everyday activities and it was reported that the positive changes in some residents were remarkable since they had arrived in the residence from the hospital. However, few of these residents had moved on to lower levels of support.

It was reported that staff perceptions of the aims and functions of community residences had changed in that they were now more often viewed as part of the rehabilitation process as opposed to a 'home for life'. During the interviews, management and clinical staff confirmed the importance of rehabilitation. They defined rehabilitation as a process of enabling the person to function at an optimal level and in as normal a social context as possible. Two catchment areas had specialised

rehabilitation teams, albeit incomplete, and could therefore provide a proactive rehabilitative role as part of community care. Within the other catchment areas, it was acknowledged that the concept of rehabilitation and recovery was very important and needed to be developed within the services. It was reported that scarcity of resources and the inefficient deployment of nursing staff led to an underdeveloped rehabilitative service. Lack of training was reported as being an important factor that inhibited rehabilitation, as the majority of the staff were trained in the philosophy of custodial care as opposed to community care.

3.8.5 Constraints on the efficient management of community residential facilities

There were a number of constraints that limited the efficient running of the community residential facilities and that inhibited the rehabilitation of the residents. These constraints were not common to all areas, although some issues were relevant on a national basis.

The issue of long-term stay charges has been an active topic of debate over the last two years. The Health Amendment Act 2005 and the Health (Charges for Inpatient Services) Regulations 2005 addressed the issue of charges for long-term institutional care. Prior to 2005, residents of community residential care were charged a weekly rent by the health services. This amount varied within and between catchment areas. However, in 2005 the Supreme Court found that there was no legal basis for the charges and consequently all HSE areas had to abolish the weekly rent contributions paid by residents. Later in the year, a repayment scheme for the refund of payments made to the health service was announced. Most of the service managers and providers reported that this caused a certain amount of upset in the residential facilities. Firstly, residents and their families were confused about the legislation. Secondly, service providers argued that the process of moving people to independent living was further impeded by the suppression of low cost accommodation previously offered in mental health residences, which limited the ability of staff to teach residents budgeting skills. In addition, one area reported that encouraging the residents to do the shopping was extremely problematic as they now had to have receipts for everything. It was felt that this further impacted on the rehabilitation process. The situation was further exacerbated when, in July 2005, new regulations which provided for different charging arrangements depending on the level of nursing care were introduced. This caused the residents and staff more distress as the maximum charge for 24-hour nursing facilities was €120 per week, or the amount of an individual's income that remained after €35 had been allowed for personal use. This left residents with little money to survive on and made it even more difficult to gather finances to secure deposits for independent accommodation. At the time of this study, the new regulations on long-stay charges had not been implemented, although residents in one area had received letters regarding charges and back payments.

Common to all 24-hour nursing facilities was the Hazard Analysis and Critical Control Points (HACCP) Health and Safety legislation. This legislation requires an analysis of risks associated with catering establishments, including commercial services and health services, and is carried out by environmental health officers. The analysis looks at operational hygiene and the implementation of these controls, identifies hazards and critical controls necessary. The situation in the majority of high support residences was that residents did not have access to the kitchen because of HACCP legislation.

Another common problem identified was the advanced age of residents who now made up a large proportion of the population in residential facilities; most of these residents had been relocated from large institutions. It was reported that the physical problems of this population outweighed the mental health problems and that these residents were much more in need of physical care rather than psychiatric intervention. A number of the residential facilities were unsuitable for those with physical disabilities. Community hospitals and homes for the elderly were not always willing to accept residents from mental health residential services, preferring instead to take those who were living alone. It was acknowledged that there was an ethical issue in moving residents to nursing homes away from their friends. In one catchment area, residential facilities for persons with learning disabilities were provided by the mental health services, yet the service did not have access to a consultant psychiatrist with a special interest in the psychiatry of learning disabilities. There was no funding for this post and services felt that this was a neglected area.

In all background interviews carried out, the issue of housing was raised. It was felt that provision of housing was not the responsibility of the mental health services and that housing should be provided by the local authority. It was highlighted that there was a possibility that the medium and low support facilities were becoming 'homes for life' as there was no alternative independent housing available for residents. As one service manager reported 'group homes were homes for the homeless until they got a house of their own'. It was reported that few residents were registered on their local housing list, although in one HSE area all residents in community accommodation were registered on the housing waiting list. However, the waiting time on that list stood at seven years and the chance of acquiring local housing was reported to be slim. All areas reported that links with local housing authorities needed to be strengthened. It was felt that, while the mental health services should not be responsible for the provision of housing, they were responsible for liaison with local authorities, voluntary groups and private landlords to ensure suitable accommodation was available. Some of the areas had already got links with voluntary groups which provided housing for those with mental health problems (e.g. Mental Health Association, Housing Association for Integrated Living, STEER), but these could be further developed.

Another issue put forward as limiting the efficient use of community residential facilities was the division of services by sector. It was reported that this limited choice for the service user. Comments included the need for more collaboration between sectors and catchment areas. Another concern was where the location of facilities that provided for an entire catchment area population. One area that serviced a large geographical area was particularly concerned about the appropriate location of services that would result in equity and accessibility for all service users.

The definition of high, medium and low support accommodation differed between and within areas and the need for a standardised definition of level of support was noted.

3.8.6 Developments for the future

Services reported that they hoped that the Mental Health Commission and the Expert Group on Mental Health Policy would provide guidelines on best practice for the management and provision of the mental health services. Issues seen as the most important included:

☐ Retraining and professional development of nursing and care staff

☐ Reorganisation of budgets for mental health care and care of the elderly

☐ Reorganisation of services to increase choice for service users

☐ Greater emphasises on rehabilitation and recovery

☐ Sufficient resources to implement and develop specialist rehabilitation and recovery mental health teams

☐ Development of the interface between mental health services and other health and social care services

☐ Best practice in the area of housing to meet the needs of those with mental health problems.

CHAPTER 4

Home Sweet Home?
Description of Community
Residences

Chapter 4
Home sweet home? Description of community residences

Chapter 4 presents the data collated from the facility questionnaires. The questionnaires were completed by the nursing officers in charge of the community residences. The researcher forwarded questionnaires to the directors of nursing in the three study areas, who forwarded them to the relevant nursing officers in community residences in the three study areas. All nursing officers in the community residences in the mental health services in the three areas completed a questionnaire (n = 102). These were then returned to the directors of nursing who forwarded them to the researcher.

The questionnaires gathered information on the demographic and diagnostic profile of residents, the numbers of residences and places in each residence, the location, and ownership of residences and the access to local services and amenities. Information was also provided on patient movement (admissions and discharges) within residences, use of respite and crisis beds, relevant exclusion criteria, waiting lists, management and policies, and, finally, food preparation.

4.1 DEMOGRAPHIC PROFILE OF RESIDENTS

There were 871 residents in the residences at the time of the study. A total of 64% (n = 554) were in high support residences,

18% (n = 153) were in medium support residences and 19% (n = 164) were in low support residences. Of the total residents 61% (n = 532) were male. A slightly higher proportion of the high support residents (60%; 333 / 554) and medium support residents (56%; 85 / 153) were male, while the majority of the low support residents (69%; 114 / 164) were female.

Almost half (47%; n = 413) of the residents were aged between 46 and 65 years. Only 21% (n = 185) were aged 45 years or under; 31% (n = 273) were aged over 65 years. Only 9% (n = 80) of residents were under the age of 35 years. Those in the high support residences had an older age profile than those in medium and low support (see Figure 4.1). There was a higher proportion of residents in high support over the age of 65 years (37%; n = 205), than in medium (20%; n = 30) or low support (23%; n = 38) and a higher proportion of those in medium support (27%; n = 42) and low support (23%; n = 38) were in the lower age range of 26 to 45 years than in high support residences (14%; n = 91).

Table 4.1 shows the diagnostic categories assigned to residents at the time of the study. Of the 871 residents, 542 (62%) had a primary diagnosis of schizophrenia.

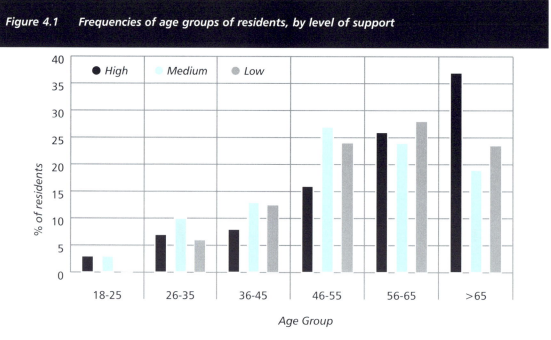

Figure 4.1   Frequencies of age groups of residents, by level of support

Table 4.1   Number (%) of residents in each diagnostic category, by level of support

	High (n = 554)	Medium (n = 153)	Low (n = 164)	Total (n = 871)
Organic	17 (3.1)	0	1 (0.06)	18 (2.1)
Schizophrenia	313 (56.5)	97 (63.3)	132 (80.5)	542 (62.2)
Other psychoses	21 (3.8)	6 (3.9)	4 (2.4)	31 (3.6)
Depression	78 (14.0)	12 (7.8)	7 (4.3)	97 (11.1)
Mania	30 (5.4)	10 (6.5)	4 (2.4)	44 (5.0)
Neurosis	11 (2.0)	2 (1.3)	2 (1.2)	15 (1.7)
Personality disorder	10 (1.8)	2 (1.3)	2 (1.2)	14 (1.6)
Alcohol disorder	15 (2.7)	2 (1.3)	4 (2.4)	21 (2.4)
Drug dependence	1 (0.01)	0	0	1 (0.01)
Intellectual disability	35 (6.3)	11 (7.2)	7 (4.3)	53 (6.1)
Unspecified	23 (4.1)	11 (7.2)	1 (0.06)	35 (4.0)
Total	554 (100.0)	153 (100.0)	164 (100.0)	871 (100.0)

The second most frequent diagnosis was depression (11%; n = 97), followed by intellectual disability (6%; n = 53) and mania (5%; n = 44). These proportions were similar across the high, medium and low support residences. As expected, few residents had a primary diagnosis of organic brain injury (2%). A total of 22 (2%) had a primary diagnosis of alcohol disorder or drug dependence. Few residents were reported as having a co-morbid alcohol (5%; n = 43) or drug (1%; n = 8) problem. A total of 35 (4%) residents had an unspecified primary diagnosis.

A small proportion of residents were reported as being in employment (21%; 181/871). Of these, 48 (5%) were in paid employment in the community and 133 (15%) were in sheltered employment. Of those in paid employment in the community, 46% (22 / 48) were in full-time employment and 54% (26 / 48) were in part-time employment.

4.2 THE PHYSICAL ENVIRONMENT OF THE COMMUNITY RESIDENCES

4.2.1 Number of residences and number of places

There was a total of 102 residences reported by the directors of nursing for the three HSE local areas, Area A (n = 39), Area B (n = 31) and Area C (n = 32). Of the total residences, 36 (35%) were high support, 25 (24%) were medium support and 41 (40%) were low support (Table 4.2). Area A provided no medium support residences and had a greater number of low support residences than Area B or Area C.

There was a total of 951 residential places in the three HSE areas. Of these, 61% (n = 584) were in high support, 18% (n = 166) were in medium support and 21% (n = 201) were in low support residences (Table 4.2).

Table 4.2   Total number (%) of residences, number (%) of residents and number (%) of places, by level of support

Level of support	Number of residences	Number of residents	Number of places
High	36 (35.3)	554 (63.6)	584 (61.4)
Medium	25 (24.6)	153 (17.6)	166 (17.5)
Low	41 (40.1)	164 (18.8)	201 (21.1)
Total	102 (100.0)	871 (100.0)	951 (100.0)

4.2.2 Location and ownership of the community residences

Almost two-thirds of the residences were situated in urban areas (70%; n = 71) or on their periphery (23%; n = 24). Significantly more of the medium (80%) and low (80%) support residences than of the high (50%) support residences were situated in urban areas (chi-square, p < 0.001). Few residences were situated in rural areas (7%; n = 7).

It was reported that the majority of the buildings housing the residences were owned by the HSE (74%; n = 76); only two were reported as leased from the local authority (one high and one medium), six were reported as owned by the voluntary sector (one high, two medium and three low) and 16 of the low support residences were reported as leased from private owners.

4.2.3 Physical environment and access to local services and amenities

As expected, high support residences had a significantly higher average number of bedrooms than medium and low support residences (Kruskal Wallis, p < 0.001; Table 4.3). Within the high support residences, there were more double rooms than single rooms. There was a similar number of double and single bedrooms in medium support residences while low support residences had more single rooms than double rooms. Only four of the residences had bedrooms with three or more beds.

The average number of bathrooms was greater in the high support residences (mean 3.89) than in medium support (mean 2.12) and low support (mean 1.44; (F (2, 101) = 13.76, p < 0.001). The ratio of residents to bathrooms was 5.96 : 1 in high support, 4.50 : 1 in medium support and 3.92 : 1 in low support. This mean ratio was significantly greater in the high support residences than in the low support residences (F = (2, 96) = 7.29, p < 0.001).

Overall, the majority of residences were unsuitable for those with mobility problems (72%). However, significantly more of the high support residences (44%) than of the medium (20%) or low support (17%) were suitable for those with mobility problems (chi square, p < 0.05). The majority provided residents with access to public phones on the premises (71%).

4.2.4 Smoking arrangements

The nursing officers reported that over half of the residences provided residents with access to a smoking room (58%). The smoking room was located outside in the majority of cases (56%). In 30% (n = 18) of the residences an inside smoking area was provided and it was reported that 14% (n = 8) had smoking rooms both inside and outside the

Table 4.3   Mean number of bedrooms in residences and standard deviations, by level of support

	High		Medium		Low	
	Mean	SD	Mean	SD	Mean	SD
Total bedrooms	9.64	5.71	5.00	1.55	3.73	1.41
Single rooms	3.81	5.44	2.44	1.50	2.59	1.55
Double rooms	4.83	3.25	2.32	1.31	1.07	0.9

Table 4.4   Mean length of time in minutes (SD) to reach other services and amenities, by level of support

	High		Medium		Low		Total
	Mean	SD	Mean	SD	Mean	SD	Mean
Time to walk to shops	11.50	11.43	9.36	4.94	6.78	5.13	9.03
Time to get to shops on public transport	9.83	10.07	7.85	4.06	6.22	3.38	7.96
Time to walk to post office	18.24	15.55	16.72	11.92	14.88	9.59	16.48
Time to post office on public transport	8.10	8.09	8.05	4.89	6.59	3.12	7.64
Time to walk to pub	11.67	11.67	9.48	9.48	8.66	8.66	9.92
Time to walk to GP surgery	21.61	21.61	17.00	17.00	14.61	14.61	17.55
Time to reach GP surgery on public transport	8.19	8.19	10.37	10.37	8.31	8.31	8.96
Time to reach day centre/hospital by minibus	36.69	38.82	27.72	34.10	15.07	20.79	25.80

residence. Of the high support residences, 89% (n = 32) provided a smoking room and 47% of these provided an indoor smoking room. A total of 48% (n = 12) of medium support and 37% (n = 15) of low support residences reported the provision of a smoking room.

4.2.5 Access to local amenities and services

Table 4.4 shows the mean length of time taken to reach local services and amenities from the residences. Time taken to walk to the shops ($F_{(2,99)} = 3.40$, $p < 0.05$) and to reach the day centre /day hospital ($F_{(2, 101)} = 4.59$, $p < 0.05$) by minibus differed significantly according to the support level of the residence. In all cases it took statistically significantly longer to reach these amenities from the high support residences than the low support residences. However these differences were small (5 – 7 minutes), except in the case of the day centres / hospitals where it took on average 20 minutes longer to reach from the high support than from the low support residences.

Few residents (4%; n = 32) had access to their own transport. Of these who had, 10 had a car, 21 had a bike and 1 had a motorbike. A total of 3% (17 / 554) of residents from high support facilities had their own transport; 5% (7 / 153) of medium support residents had their own, as had 5% (8 / 164) of residents from low support residences.

Table 4.5	Number (%) of admissions in the last three years (2002 – 2004), by level of support			
	High	**Medium**	**Low**	**Total**
Less than 6 months prior to the study	89 *(24.8)*	34 *(22.4)*	14 *(36.8)*	137 *(24.9)*
6 – 12 months prior to the study	79 *(22.0)*	34 *(22.4)*	9 *(23.7)*	122 *(22.2)*
13 – 36 months prior to the study	191 *(53.2)*	84 *(55.2)*	15 *(39.5)*	290 *(52.8)*
Total	359 *(65.4)*	152 *(27.7)*	38 *(6.9)*	549 *(100.0)*

Table 4.6	Total number of residents discharged and place discharged to, by level of support			
	High	**Medium**	**Low**	**Total**
Higher support	36 *(26.7)*	7 *(33.3)*	5 *(21.8)*	48 *(26.8)*
Same level of support	5 *(3.7)*	2 *(9.5)*	5 *(21.8)*	12 *(6.7)*
Lower support	27 *(20.0)*	5 *(24.0)*	1 *(4.3)*	33 *(18.4)*
Home / family	56 *(41.5)*	7 *(33.3)*	7 *(30.4)*	70 *(39.1)*
General hospital	8 *(6.0)*	0	3 *(13.0)*	11 *(6.1)*
Hospice / nursing home	3 *(2.2)*	0	2 *(8.7)*	5 *(2.8)*
Total	135 *(100.0)*	21 *(100.0)*	23 *(100.0)*	179 *(100.0)*

A total of 28% of the residences had access to a minibus (i.e. 47% of the high support residences, 24% of the medium support residences and 15% of the low support residences). All the medium and low support residences shared the minibus with other residences, while only 35% of the high support residences did so.

4.3 ADMISSIONS AND DISCHARGES

Table 4.5 shows the number and proportion of admissions to the high, medium and low support residences in the three years prior to data collection (2002 – 2004). A total of 137 admissions to the residences was reported for the last six months, with the majority of these being to high support residences (65%; n = 89). The highest number of admissions was to the high support units, with 359 residents being admitted over a period of 36

months. The year prior to the study a total of 259 admissions were reported.

Regarding discharges in the year prior to data collection for the study (2004), there was a total of 179 discharges. These discharges were reported for a total of 61% of the residences (26% high, 15% medium, 20% low). Table 4.6 shows the number of discharges and place of discharge of the residents. The majority of these were from high support residences (75%; n = 135) with few from medium (12%; n = 21) or low (13%; n = 23) support residences. Of the total, 39% were discharged home or to family. A total of 27% (n = 48) were discharged to a higher support level, while 7% (n = 12) were discharged to the same level of support and 18% (n = 33) to a lower level of support. Only two residents were discharged to nursing homes and three were discharged to a hospice. A total of 11 residents were discharged to a general

Table 4.7   Number (%) of residences employing exclusion criteria and the specific exclusion criteria employed, by level of support

	High (n = 36)	Medium (n = 25)	Low (n = 41)	Total (n = 102)
Applying any exclusion criteria	29 (80.6)	10 (40.0)	26 (63.4)	65 (63.7)
Excluding acute psychotic disorders	19 (52.8)	2 (8.0)	17 (41.5)	38 (37.3)
Excluding substance abuse	9 (25.0)	2 (8.0)	2 (4.9)	13 (12.7)
Excluding alcohol abuse	11 (30.6)	7 (28.0)	8 (19.5)	26 (25.5)
Excluding severe physical disease	22 (61.1)	7 (28.0)	23 (56.1)	52 (51.0)
Excluding organic brain disease	19 (52.8)	6 (64.0)	23 (56.1)	48 (47.1)
Excluding intellectual disability	9 (25.0)	6 (24.0)	11 (26.8)	26 (25.5)
Excluding violent behaviours	14 (38.9)	7 (28.0)	13 (31.7)	34 (33.3)
Excluding former CMH patient	7 (19.4)	2 (8.0)	9 (22.0)	18 (17.6)

hospital. Over a quarter (27%) of the discharges from high support residences were to higher levels of support. Although the questionnaire did not specify to which unit the discharges went, it may be assumed that a higher level of support for those in a high support residence would be an inpatient facility. One-third of those from medium support and 22% of those discharged from low support went to higher levels of support. Nearly half of the high support discharges went home or to family (41%), while 33% of those discharged from medium support and 30% of those discharged from low support were discharged home or to family.

4.4   USE OF PLACES, EXCLUSION CRITERIA AND WAITING LISTS

4.4.1 Respite and crisis beds

Of the total 951 places (beds) in the residences, 55 were designated as respite beds (n = 46) or crisis beds (n = 9). The nursing officers reported that these beds were provided in 29% (31 / 102) of the residences. The majority of the respite beds were in high support (37 / 46) as were the majority of

crisis beds (7 / 9). It was also reported that a total of 21% (21 / 102) of the residences had beds that had been used to accommodate transfers from acute units due to bed shortages. Again the majority of these beds were in high support residences (16 / 21). Of the total number having designated respite beds (n = 24), 17 had policies regarding the use of such beds. Of the total number of residences having designated crisis beds (n = seven), four had related policies. Only five of the residences had policies relating to the use of beds for transfers from acute units.

4.4.2 Exclusion criteria and waiting lists

The questionnaire provided a list of possible exclusion criteria for admission to the residences and respondents were asked to indicate which ones applied in their case. In 64% one or more of the exclusion criteria for admission to the residences were employed (Table 4.7). The majority of high support (81%) and low support (63%) residences employed exclusion criteria, as did 40% of the medium support. Severe physical disease

(51%) and organic brain disease (47%) were the most frequently employed exclusion criteria. Over one-third of the residences reported that they employed criteria excluding those with substance and / or alcohol abuse problems (38%) or violent behaviours (33%).

A total of 31% of high, 32% of medium and 5% of low support residences had waiting lists for placements. Only two of the residences reported estimated waiting time for a place in the residence. These waiting times were six weeks and twelve weeks.

4.5 MANAGEMENT AND POLICES

4.5.1 Placement rights

The nursing officers of the residences were asked who had ownership of beds (placement rights), referring to who had responsibility for admissions and discharges to the residences. The nursing officers reported that the placement rights lay with the HSE local area in 12% of the residences. A total of 34% of the nursing officers specifically stated that the placement rights lay with the consultant psychiatrist. A large proportion of the placement rights were regarded as being with the rehabilitation team (31%; n = 32) while 13% of the nursing officers reported that the placement rights lay with the sector team. In only one instance was it reported that placement rights lay with the acute hospital, and 9% reported that the placement rights lay with the social support team.

4.5.2 Assessment

Just over half of the residences (55%) had carried out a formal assessment of residents prior to admission, while 27% had an informal assessment and 14% had no assessment procedure. The question was not answered in 4% of the residences. Over half of the high

(53%) and medium (84%) support residences, and 39% of the low support residences had a formal assessment procedure. Of the high support residences, 44% performed informal assessments of the residents, while 4% of the medium and 27% of the low support residences had such an assessment prior to admission. One high support facility (3%) had no assessment procedure and 13 (32%) of the low support residences had no assessment procedure. All of the medium support residences that answered the question reported having assessments (3 did not answer).

4.5.3 Staff meetings

In half of the residences, there were no planned formal staff meetings (51%). A total of 44% of medium and 71% of low support residences had no formal staff meetings. However, the majority of the high support residences had planned formal meetings for staff (72%). The nursing officers reported that the majority of the residences had staff meetings to discuss the treatment provided to residents and response to treatment (81%). Over half of the residences (52%) did not have planned meetings open to residents to discuss the organisation and procedures of the residence. Few residences had planned meetings with relatives (15%).

4.5.4 Quality monitoring

A total of 27% of the residences had an evaluation and review plan for monitoring of the services. Regarding evaluation of the quality services and management in the residences, only 22% of the residences used performance indicators to evaluate the service, 23% logged surveillance of problematic situations, 19% monitored residents' satisfaction and 17% monitored family satisfaction.

4.5.5 Health and safety

Table 4.8   *Number (%) of residences that had polices on health and safety and related matters, by level of support*

	High (n = 36)	Medium (n = 25)	Low (n = 41)	Total (n = 102)
Dangerous situations	35 (97.2)	22 (88.0)	35 (85.4)	92 (90.2)
Health and safety policy	36 (100)	16 (64.0)	26 (63.4)	78 (76.5)
Electronic fire alarm	36 (100)	23 (92.0)	39 (95.1)	98 (96.1)
Intervention programmes	22 (61.1)	7 (28.0)	4 (9.8)	33 (32.4)
Resident and family feedback	20 (55.6)	6 (24.0)	22 (53.7)	48 (47.1)
FOI / Protection act information	24 (66.7)	16 (64.0)	34 (82.9)	74 (72.5)
Emergency telephone numbers	24 (66.7)	23 (92.0)	37 (90.2)	84 (82.4)
Information pack for residents	17 (47.2)	13 (52.0)	15 (36.6)	45 (44.1)

The majority of residences had policies in place regarding health and safety issues (Table 4.8). Few had information on treatment intervention programmes (32.4%) or resident and family feedback (47%). Over half of the high support residences had information on intervention programmes (61%) and obtained resident and family feedback (56%). Less than half of the high (47%) and low (37%) support residences provided information packs for residents, while only 52% of medium support residences provided such packs.

4.5.6 Rules and regulations

Table 4.9 shows the number of residences where rules and regulations were imposed on the residents. The table shows that there was little difference between the three levels of support in the frequency with which rules and regulations were employed in relation to unsupervised leave, locking of the bathroom door, unscheduled visiting hours and unscheduled bedtimes.

4.5.6.1 Leaving the residence

In the high support residences, staff supervised the daytime comings and goings of the residents and in only 22% were residents provided with front door keys. Bedtime checks were carried out in all high support residences and 86% required residents to notify staff if they were going out, compared with 64% of medium and 10% of low support residences. It is interesting to note that, while low support residences were not staffed, a small proportion appeared to restrict residents' activities. For example, in 10% of low support residences the comings and goings of residents were supervised, while in 71% residents were required to be up at a certain time during weekdays. Furthermore, in 10% it was reported that residents were required to inform staff where they were going.

---

2   One question, relating to problems with living conditions, was omitted as irrelevant to the study.

Table 4.9   *Number (%) of residences that imposed rules and regulations concerning freedom within the residences, by level of support*

	High (n = 36)	Medium (n = 25)	Low (n = 41)	Total (n = 102)
Supervised daytime comings and going (yes)	36 (100)	5 (20.0)	4 (9.8)	45 (44.1)
Unsupervised leave (yes)	34 (94.4)	23 (92.0)	41 (100)	98 (96.1)
Front door key (yes)	8 (22.2)	22 (88.0)	41 (100)	71 (69.6)
Lock bathroom (yes)	29 (80.6)	22 (88.0)	41 (100)	92 (90.2)
Scheduled visiting hours for visitors (yes)	2 (5.6)	3 (12.0)	1 (2.4)	6 (5.9)
Scheduled bedtime for residents (no)	29 (80.6)	20 (80.0)	41 (100)	90 (88.2)
Bedtime checks by staff (yes)	36 (100)	21 (84.0)	2 (4.9)	59 (57.8)
Residents had to be up at certain time during weekdays (yes)	33 (91.7)	20 (80.0)	29 (70.7)	82 (80.4)
Residents had to be up at certain time during be up weekends/ holidays (yes)	12 (33.3)	2 (8.0)	1 (2.4)	15 (14.7)
Residents informed staff where they are going (yes)	31 (86.1)	16 (64.0)	4 (9.8)	51 (50.0)
Residents check in at certain time (yes)	20 (55.6)	14 (56.0)	4 (9.8)	38 (37.3)

4.5.6.2 Bedroom use and privacy

Table 4.10 shows the number of residences where rules and regulations concerning bedroom use and privacy were imposed. Regarding privacy, it was reported in the majority of community residences that residents had access to their own space (86% of high, 100% of medium and 93% of low support residences). Nursing officers reported that only a few of the residences allowed residents the choice of single rooms, although 68% of low support residences were able to provide residents with the choice of single rooms. As Table 4.3 shows, the sharing of rooms was most likely due to the lack of single rooms in the residences. The majority of residents had to share a room, yet in only 58% of high, 12% of medium and 49% of low support residences were residents given the choice of whom to share the room with. Again, this was most likely a result of the inability of residences to provide residents with a choice of type of room. Residents were allowed in bedrooms during the day in over half of the residences, but it was reported that this was not encouraged. It was reported, that in 61% of the low support residences, residents were able to lock the bedroom doors; in only 19% of the high and 28% of the medium support residences were residents allowed to do so. Again,

Table 4.10   Number (%) of residences that had rules and regulations concerning bedroom use and privacy, by level of support

	High (n = 36)	Medium (n = 25)	Low (n = 41)	Total (n = 102)
Residents stay in bedrooms during daytime (yes)	22 (61.1)	12 (48.0)	26 (63.4)	60 (58.8)
Can residents lock bedroom? (yes)	7 (19.4)	7 (28.0)	25 (61.0)	39 (38.2)
Can residents smoke in bedrooms? (yes)	1 (2.8)	1 (2.8)	8 (19.5)	10 (9.8)
Do residents have their own space? (yes)	31 (86.1)	25 (100)	38 (92.7)	94 (92.2)
Can residents choose whom to share room with? (yes)	21 (58.3)	3 (12.0)	20 (48.8)	44 (43.1)
Can residents choose single rooms? (yes)	11 (30.6)	5 (20.0)	28 (68.3)	44 (43.1)

this could have been a feature of shared rooms as opposed to a restriction on access to bedrooms. As expected, the nursing officers reported that less than 3% of high or medium support residences allowed residents to smoke in the bedrooms, as compared to 20% of the low support residences.

4.5.6.3 Restrictiveness

In order to assess the overall characteristics of the social climate of the residences a restrictiveness score was composed by the researcher using the 22 items on the questionnaire dealing with the internal rules of the residence. The researcher scored each item as '0' (absent) or '1' (present). Restrictiveness scores could range from 0 - 22, with higher scores indicating a higher degree of restrictiveness. The mean restrictiveness score was significantly different in the three levels of support ($F_{(2,101)} = 70.94$, $p < 0.001$), with the high support being more restrictive. The mean restrictiveness score for high support was 11.0, while for medium it was 8.4 and low was 3.8.

4.5.7 Food

Table 4.11 shows who had responsibility for the preparation of the resident's food. A quarter of both high support (25%) and low support (24%) residences had their food prepared by kitchen staff in a psychiatric unit or hospital. Kitchen staff prepared the food in the majority of high support residences (58%), while the staff and residents prepared the food in the majority of the medium support residences (52%). Care staff and residents (44%) or residents themselves (39%) prepared the food in the low support residences.

4.6   SUMMARY

The majority of the residents were 46 years of age or over at the time of the study. One-third were over the age of 65 years. The age profile in the high support residences was older than that in the medium and low support, and the youngest age profile was in the medium support residences. The majority of the residents had a primary diagnosis of schizophrenia. A very small proportion of residents were employed either in the community or in sheltered employment.

Table 4.11   Number (%) of residences and the responsibility for food preparation, by level of support

	High (n = 36)	Medium (n = 25)	Low (n = 41)	Total (n = 102)
Psychiatric hospital kitchen staff	9 (25.0)	1 (4.0)	10 (24.4)	20 (19.6)
Residents	1 (2.8)	5 (20.0)	16 (39.0)	22 (21.6)
Staff	1 (2.8)	5 (20.0)	4 (9.8)	10 (9.8)
Staff and residents	11 (30.6)	13 (52.0)	18 (43.9)	42 (41.2)
Kitchen staff	21 (58.3)	1 (4.0)	3 (7.3)	25 (24.5)
Staff, kitchen staff, residents	2 (5.6)	1 (4.0)	0	3 (2.9)

The data presented here detail the provision of all community residences in the three study areas. On average, high support residences provided 16.2 (SD 7.76) places per residence, medium support residences provided 6.9 (SD 2.24) places and low support residences provided 4.90 (SD 1.94) places. There was a total of 951 places with over half in high support (60%), one-fifth in low support (21%) and only 16% in medium support. Not all the places were occupied at the time of the study, with only 871 people in the residences. This resulted in 80 empty places, although there were 55 designated respite or crisis places and 21 residences reported having to use places for transfers from acute units, making a total of 76 such places. The issue of whether places in community residences should be used for these purposes is discussed in Chapter 10. Very few single rooms were available in high support residences, with slightly more available in medium and low support residences. There was a higher ratio of residents to bathrooms in high support residences than in medium or low support.

The majority of the residences were situated in urban areas and were owned by the HSE. The length of time taken to walk from the community residences to local amenities such as the shops, post office or GP was, on average, less than 20 minutes. However, the time taken to reach the day hospital or day centre from the community residences by transport was, on average, over half an hour for those in high support. Very few of the residents had their own transport, while just over a quarter of the facilities had access to a minibus. Less than half of the high support residences had access to a minibus and, of those that had, just over one-third of the residences shared the minibus with other residences.

A total of 259 admissions and 179 discharges were reported for the 12 months prior to the study. The majority of these related to high support residences.

Over half of the community residences reported that they employed one or more criteria for excluding potential residents. The exclusion criteria most frequently reported were severe physical disease and organic brain disorder. It was reported that a large proportion of the residences tended to exclude those who might have been more difficult to treat (i.e. substance and alcohol abusers and those with violent behaviours).

Waiting lists were reported for approximately one-third of the high and medium support residences, while a much lower proportion of the low support residences reported waiting lists. The approximate time on the waiting list was not reported for the majority of residences.

While over half of the residences a formal assessment procedure was reported to be in operation, few had planned meetings that involved staff and residents or residents' families. The majority had polices regarding health and safety, dangerous situations, freedom of information and emergency telephone numbers. However, few had polices in place that concerned intervention programmes or feedback from residents and families.

The results suggested that the high support facilities were the most restrictive in terms of the internal rules of the residence. This was followed by the medium support facilities, with the low support residences the least restrictive.

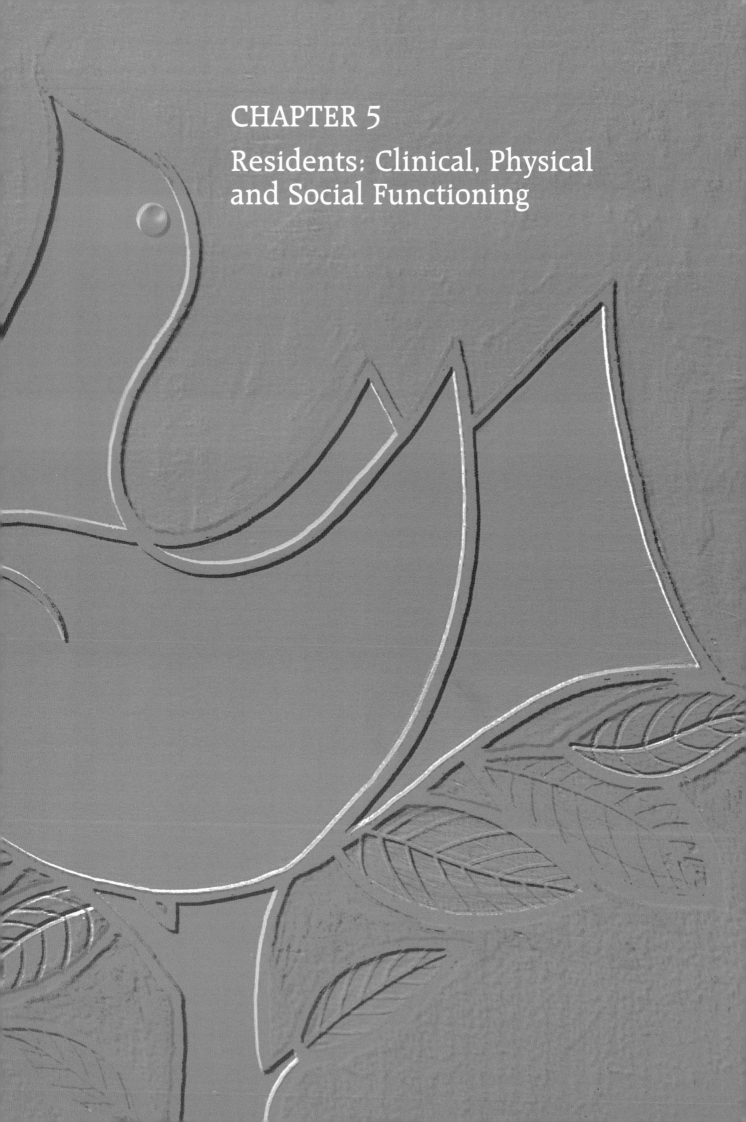

CHAPTER 5

Residents: Clinical, Physical
and Social Functioning

Chapter 5

Residents: clinical, physical and social functioning

We now pass from description of the entire number of residents (871) to the sample of 138 who were interviewed. We begin with a review of the demographic, clinical and functional characteristics of these 138 residents and continue with a review of the perceived appropriateness of their placement. Clinical status and functioning are then presented on the basis of data obtained by the researcher by means of the key-worker questionnaire and the residents themselves (through self-report Disability Assessment Scale II (DAS II)).

5.1 DEMOGRAPHIC AND CLINICAL CHARACTERISTICS OF THE SAMPLE

5.1.1 Demography

A sample of 138 residents was interviewed for the study, comprising 16% of the total residents in the three participating areas (138 / 871). Of these, 59% (n = 82) were from high support residences, 18% (n = 25) were from medium support residences and 22% (n = 31) were from low support residences. This compares to 64% of high support residents, 18% of medium support residents and 19% of low support residents in all community residential facilities in the three study areas.

There was no significant gender difference in the sample (males 49%, females 51%; p > 0.05), nor was there any significant gender difference, by level of support (p > 0.05). There was a slightly lower proportion of males than females in the sample interviewed (49%) as opposed to the total residents reported for all residences (61%) in the area.

The mean age of the sample was 53.7 years (SD 13.4). The age range was 22 to 88 years and there was no significant difference in the mean ages between high (mean 53.7 years, SD 12.5), medium (mean 58.2 years, SD 13.3) and low (mean 50.16 years, SD 15.1) support.

The largest proportion of the sample was aged between 46 and 65 years (57%). Only 24% (n = 33) of the residents were under the age of 45 years. A total of 22% (n = 31) were over the age of 65 years while 9% (n = 13) were under the age of 35 years. Of those in the high support residences, 22% were over the age of 65 years, compared with 28% in medium support and 19% in low support residences. The age profile of the sample of residents interviewed was very similar to that reported for all 871 residents. In both groups a large proportion of the residents were between the ages of 46 and 65 years (47% versus 57%). Only a small proportion in both groups were under the age of 35 years (both 9%).

A large proportion of the sample were single (87%), with 3% married and 10% separated or divorced. Few had post-secondary or third-level education (22%); however, 46% had attended secondary school.

Not unexpectedly a total of 40% of the sample were unemployed. Only 2% were employed full time and only 5% were employed part time. A total of 27% were in sheltered employment. This gives a total of 34% of the sampled residents in sheltered or paid employment. A total of 25% of the sample were in training, on courses or retired. Comparisons with information from all residents in residential facilities would suggest that a greater proportion of those sampled were employed. For example, 5% of all residents were reported as being in paid employment and 15% were reported as being in sheltered employment.

5.1.2 Psychiatric history

The duration of illness ranged from 3 to 62 years, with a mean duration of 26.6 years. The age of first contact with services ranged from 15 to 70 years, with a mean age of 26.3 years. The length of time that the residents had lived in their current accommodation ranged from 0.5 to 25 years, with an overall mean of 6.8 years. One-way ANOVA on the mean length of time the resident had lived in the current accommodation showed that those in medium support residences had been there significantly longer (mean 8.52 years) than those in high (mean 5.2 years) or low (mean 6.8 years) support residences (F (2, 137) = 3.89, p < 0.05). Despite these relatively lengthy periods of residence, there was significant movement in and out of the residences, as evidenced by the number of admissions in the past 12 months as detailed in Section 4.3.

The majority of the residents had had periods of inpatient hospitalisations (97%) in psychiatric units or hospitals. Hospitalisation while a resident was greatest for those in low support (42%), while only 27% of high and 20% of medium support residents were hospitalised while a resident. A large proportion of the sample had no hospital admissions in the last five years (64%), with a greater proportion of the medium support (82%) than the high (61%) or low (59%) support residents having had no admissions. For those who had inpatient hospitalisations in the last five years, the average number of admissions was 2.6. There was no significant difference (p > 0.05) between the average number of hospitalisations for residents in high (mean 3.0), medium (mean 1.7) and low (mean 1.8) support residences.

Regarding the course of illness in the last five years, only 9% of the residents had an absence of symptoms. These included 5% of high support, 20% of medium support and 13% of low support. Remission with intermittent episodes over the last five years was evident in 5% of the residents, while partial remission was evident in 16%. The most commonly reported course of illness in the last five years for high (66%), medium (60%) and low (52%) support residents was

symptoms that were persistent, but stable. Only 3% of the residents were reported as having progressive deterioration.

5.2 CLINICAL, SOCIAL AND PHYSICAL FUNCTIONING AND LEVEL OF DISABILITY IN EVERYDAY LIVING ACTIVITIES

5.2.1 Clinical functioning

5.2.1.1 Level of symptoms

The Brief Psychiatric Rating Scale (BPRS) was completed by the researcher at the interview with the resident. The scale was used to measure the psychopathology of the residents over the two weeks prior to interview. The 24 symptoms measured are rated on a seven-point scale (i.e. 1 = no symptoms, 7= extremely severe symptoms). The total scores on the BPRS can range from 24 (no symptoms present) to 168 (extremely severe in all symptoms). The average BPRS score was 35.8 (range 24 – 76) for high support residents, 30.2 (range 24 – 45) for medium support residents and 30.3 (range 24 – 45) for low support residents indicating that BPRS mean scores for all groups were in the mild category. Not surprisingly however there were significant group differences, with those from low support residences having a significantly lower score than those from high support residences (F (2, 128) = 8.96, p = 0.01).

5.2.1.2 Global functioning

The Global Assessment of Functioning Scale (GAF) provided a measure of the clinician's judgement of the individual's overall current level of functioning. It takes into consideration psychological, social and occupational functioning on a hypothetical continuum of mental health– illness. Each individual was rated on a scale of 0 – 100, with higher scores indicating superior functioning. The mean score of the high support residents (55.37; range 20 – 90) fell within the moderate symptom range *(moderate symptoms or moderate difficulty in social or occupational functioning)*, while the mean scores for the residents in medium support (66.84; range 35 - 95) and in low support (61.94; range 25– 85) fell within the mild symptoms range (*some mild symptoms or some difficulty in social or occupational functioning, but generally functioning pretty well and has some meaningful interpersonal relationships*). There was a significant difference in mean GAF scores between the levels of support (F (2, 137) = 4.92, p < 0.01). The high support group scored significantly lower than the medium and low support groups, with the medium support residents having the highest level of functioning.

5.2.1.3 Psychopathology and disability

The Health of the Nation Outcome Scale (HoNOS) was designed to assess psychopathology and disability in the two weeks prior to interview. It is a 12-item scale measuring clinical and social functioning and is rated on a five-point scale (0 – 4), with 3 – 4 indicating significant or severe problems.[2] Total scores on the HoNOS used in this study can range from 0 – 44. Table 5.1 shows the percentage of residents in each of the categories for each individual item.

Total scores were computed for residents and subjected to a Kruskal Wallis Test. Analysis on the total HoNOS scores yielded significant group differences (p < 0.001). Those in high support residences had higher mean scores (11.9; range 0 - 30) than those in medium (5.6; range 0 - 17) or in low support (6.2; range 0 - 26).

5.2.2 Physical Health Index

The Physical Health Index (PHI) was used to measure the physical health of the sample of residents and was comprised of eight items. This was completed by the key workers. This questionnaire asked about physical health disabilities in eight domains and was rated on a four-point scale from 0 – 3. Total scores on the PHI can range from 0 – 24. Table 5.2 summarises the results on each of the PHI items. As can be seen, and contrary to expectations given the age and clinical profile, a few residents were experiencing moderate to severe health problems with the majority experiencing no disabilities. The mean scores for the three groups were 1.79 (range 0 – 13) for high support residents, 0.80 (range 0 – 5) for medium support residents and 1.06 (range 0 – 6) for low support residents. A one-way ANOVA comparing the mean scores was not significant (p > 0.05).

Table 5.1   Percentage of residents in each category of the HoNOS individual items

Item	No problem	Minor / mild	Moderate / severe
Overactive, aggressive, disruptive or agitated behaviour	65.9	21.0	11.6
Non-accidental self-injury	95.7	2.2	0.7
Problem drinking or drug taking	84.1	14.5	0.7
Cognitive problems	42.0	38.4	17.4
Physical illness or disability problems	60.9	27.5	10.8
Problems associated with hallucinations and delusions	47.8	34.0	16.6
Problems with depressed mood	47.8	44.2	6.5
Other mental and behavioural problems	47.8	34.0	14.4
Problems with relationships	44.9	39.1	15.2
Problems with activities of daily living	33.3	38.4	26.8
Problems with occupation and activities	37.0	34.0	26.1

5.2.3 Functioning in the last thirty days

The WHO Disability Assessment Scale (DAS II) is a measure of functioning and disability. The scale is a 12-item questionnaire and each item is rated on a five point scale from 0 – 4. Total scores can range from 0 – 48 with a lower score indicating less disability. It assesses functioning and disabilities in the last 30 days. The domains of functioning assessed by the DAS II include understanding and communicating, getting around, self care, getting along with others, household and work activities and participation in society. Two DAS II questionnaires were employed in the current study. One was completed by the key worker for the resident and one was based on the self

Table 5.2   Percentage of residents experiencing physical health disabilities

Disability	No disability	Mild disability	Moderate disability	Severe disability
Cardiovascular	84.1	10.1	5.8	0
Respiratory	85.5	5.8	8.7	0
Digestive	83.3	11.6	4.3	0.7
Urogential	92.0	2.2	4.3	1.4
Motor	89.1	5.8	4.3	0.7
Central nervous system	87.0	6.5	6.5	0
Metabolic / endocrine system	82.6	9.4	7.2	0.7
Infective system (including HIV)	100	0	0	0

report of the residents. Thus two DAS II questionnaires were completed for every resident. This allowed comparison between the resident's perception of their own functioning and the key worker's perception of the functioning of the resident. There was a significant positive correlation, albeit weak, between resident's total DAS II scores and the key worker's rating of the resident (Pearson's r = 0.314, p < 0.001). However, it is important to note that while there was a significant correlation between the scores, the total mean scores differed between the residents' and the key workers' ratings (t (237.3) = -5.43, p < 0.001). The total mean score for the residents' ratings was 6.35 (range 0 – 34) and the total mean score provided by the key workers was 12.51 (range 0 – 46). Kruskal Wallis Tests on both scores yielded significant differences between residents in high, medium and low support residences (resident ratings p < 0.01; key worker ratings (p < 0.001). In both analyses, not unexpectedly, the high support residents had greater mean scores suggesting that they experienced greater disability than the medium and low support residents.

5.3   APPROPRIATENESS OF PLACEMENT

The key workers were asked to indicate whether they thought the resident was appropriately placed in the residence at the time of the study. Of all residents, 85% were reported as being appropriately placed and 2% of the residents' key workers reported that they were unsure of the appropriateness of placement. A total of 17 (13%) residents were reported by key workers as being inappropriately placed. Of these, ten were in high support residences, two were in medium support residences and five were in low support residences. Only three residents (one each in high, medium and low residences) were reported as being more appropriately

placed in independent living. It was reported that four would be better placed in an independent group home (two high and two low support residents) and four (two high and two low support residents) would be better placed in a medium support home. A total of two residents would be better placed in a higher support (one high and one medium support resident) and another two would be better placed in a nursing home (two high support residents). The main barrier to appropriate placement was unavailable facilities (n = 8), while three reported that a facility was available but had a waiting list. The mental state of the resident was reported as the precluding discharge of three of the residents inappropriately placed. In two of the inappropriately placed residents, the resident's relatives had refused transfers and in one the doctor's opinion was considered to have been a barrier to appropriate placement.

The key workers were asked where they saw the resident living in six months time. A total of 88% of the key workers reported that the residents would be living in the same residences. Only six residents were predicted to be living in lower support and only two were predicted as living in independent accommodation.

5.4   SUMMARY

A total of 138 residents participated in the interview stage of the study. This sample was 16% of the total number of residents in the three study areas. The majority of the participating sample of residents were from high support residences (59%), while 18% were from medium support and 22% from low support. The sample of residents interviewed was representative of those in all the residences in terms of gender and age. The employment question for the sample of residents interviewed enquired as to whether the resident was in training, education or retired while the question for the nursing officers only sought the total number of residents in sheltered or paid employment. When looking at the proportions in sheltered and paid employment, the results for all residents in the residences and the residents that were interviewed were similar for paid employment. For example, 7% of the sample interviewed was in paid employment compared to 5% of all residents in the residences. Of the residents interviewed, 27% were in sheltered employment compared to 15% of the total sample.

The duration of illness among the residents interviewed ranged from three to sixty-two years. The average duration of illness was 26 years and the average age at first contact with services was 26 years. The residents had lived in their current accommodation for an average of seven years. Residents in the medium support residences were significantly longer in their current accommodation than those in high or low support. Notwithstanding the statistical significance of the result, there was little difference in the average length of time in the current accommodation, with a difference of approximately three years from the highest average length of time to the lowest. The majority of the residents had had previous hospitalisations, but a smaller percentage had had inpatient hospitalisations in the previous five years. Only a few of the residents were reported as having an absence of symptoms in the previous five years. Of those who had symptoms, for the majority the symptoms were persistent, but stable. This is in line with findings regarding current symptoms where the resident's mean score indicated that symptoms were present, but mild. The majority of the residents were judged by key worker as being appropriately placed at the time of the study. Of those who were inappropriately placed, it was reported that the majority would be better placed in independent group homes or in medium support residences. The main barriers perceived by key workers to appropriate placement were unavailability of appropriate facilities. Furthermore, key workers predicted that the majority of residents would be in the same accommodation in six months' time.

There was a significant difference in the overall current level of functioning of the residents between high, medium and low

support residences, with residents from high support having poorer functioning to those in medium or low support. The residents in high support were reported as having moderate difficulties in social or occupational functioning, while those in medium and low support were reported as having mild difficulties.

Regarding clinical and social functioning in the previous two weeks, the majority of the residents were reported by key workers as having no problems. An exception to this was in relation to activities of daily living. Over one-third of the residents were reported as having mild problems and over a quarter were reported as having moderate to severe difficulties. There was a significant difference between the groups on the total score, indicating that the high support residents had poorer functioning to those in medium and low support.

The majority of residents were reported by the key workers as having no current physical health problems and there was no significant difference between the physical health functioning of residents in high, medium and low support residences.

Functioning and disability in relation to communication, self-care, social contacts, activities and participation in society over the last month were rated by key workers and by the residents themselves. The results showed that overall, the key workers rated the residents' functioning as lower than that provided by the resident's themselves. There was weak significant positive correlation between the scores, demonstrating that the higher the resident's rating of functioning, the higher the key worker's rating also. The residents in high support were reported, both by the key workers and by themselves, as functioning at a lower level than those in medium or low support.

In most areas the high support residents were functioning at a significantly lower level than the medium and low support residents although the extent to which this lower level of functioning would affect independent living is questionable. For example, the findings highlighted that the majority of the residents were experiencing few problems in clinical, physical and social functioning and it was only in the activities of daily living that mild to moderate problems were evident. Yet the key workers judged the majority of residents to be appropriately placed, whether in high, medium or low support facilities. This anomaly causes some concern and would suggest that the care provided to residents in community residences may over-provide for their needs.

CHAPTER 6
Citizenship: Social Support,
Community Integration and
Rights

Chapter 6

Citizenship: social support, community integration and rights

This chapter provides information on the sample of 138 residents relating to their status as citizens, as supplied by key workers and residents and, in the case of rights, by the facilities questionnaire.

6.1 SOCIAL SUPPORT, INDEPENDENCE AND COMMUNITY INTEGRATION

6.1.1 Social support

The social support network of the residents was assessed by the self-reports of the residents and by asking the key worker questions regarding visits to family and friends and the system of support provided to the resident in the last year.

Table 6.1 presents the key workers' reported system of support (i.e. family and friends) for the residents in high, medium and low levels of support over the last year. A total of 38% were perceived to have family and friends who were interested and willing to provide support. The key workers reported that 24% of residents had a support system available, but that family and friends had doubts about their ability to provide support. The key workers reported that 11% of the residents had family and friends with the potential to provide support, but that they had severe difficulties in putting this into action. It was reported that a total of 28% of the residents had no family or friends to provide support.

Key workers were asked to indicate whether the residents had visits from family and friends or if the residents went to visit family and friends. A total of 72% of high, 56% of medium and 55% of low support residents had visits from family and friends to the residence, while 68% of high, 76% of medium and 84% of low support residents visited family and friends in their own homes.

The residents' self-reported social support network was assessed in four domains – everyday psychological support, everyday instrumental support, instrumental crisis support and psychological crisis support. Examples of these social support domains include:

- Everyday psychological support – whom do you like to do everyday things with?

- Everyday instrumental support - whom do you turn to when you need a small favour?

- Instrumental crisis support – whom would you discuss an important decision with?

- Psychological crisis support – whom would you turn to if you wanted to talk to someone during an upsetting time?

Residents were asked to indicate whether they would use social support networks (i.e. nursing or care staff, other residents or family and friends from outside the residence) in the above scenarios and, if so, whom would they ask for help. Figure 6.1 shows the percentage of residents who would seek help from others in each

Table 6.1	Key workers' reported system of support for residents (number (%)) in the last year			
	High (n = 82)	Medium (n = 25)	Low (n = 31)	Total (n = 138)
Family / friends interested and willing to provide support	27 (32.9)	12 (48.0)	13 (41.9)	52 (37.7)
Family / friends have doubts about ability to provide support	18 (22.0)	6 (24.0)	9 (29.0)	33 (23.9)
Potential to provide support but severe difficulties putting into action	13 (15.9)	1 (4.0)	1 (3.2)	15 (10.9)
Absence of family / friends to provide support	24 (29.3)	6 (24.0)	8 (25.8)	38 (27.5)
Total	82 (100.0)	25 (100.0)	31 (100.0)	138 (100.0)

Figure 6.1   Resident's reported social support network in four domains

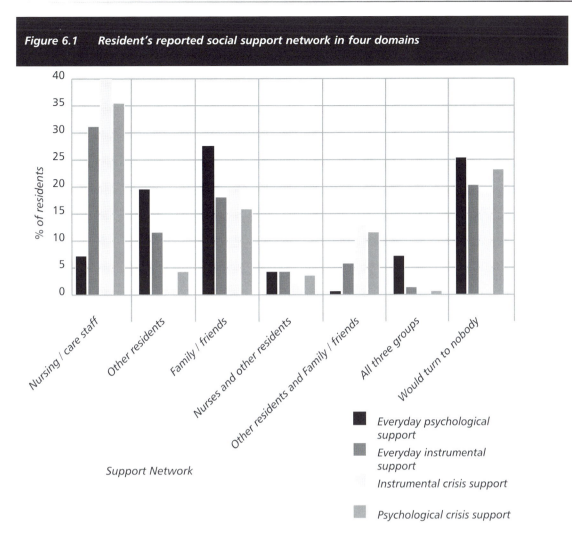

Everyday psychological
support

Everyday instrumental
support

Instrumental crisis support

Psychological crisis support

of the social support domains. This shows that support was sought from only nursing and care staff most often for everyday instrumental support, instrumental crisis support and psychological crisis support. Only family and friends or only other residents were most often reported as providing everyday psychological support. All three groups of support networks together (i.e. staff, family or friends and other residents) were seldom sought for support. A total of 25% of residents reported that they had no one to do everyday things with (everyday psychological support). Likewise, 23% reported that there was no one to whom they would turn to during times of psychological need (psychological crisis support). A total of 20% reported that they would not ask anyone to do a favour for them (everyday instrumental support) and 18% reported that would not ask anyone for support if they had to make an important decision (instrumental crisis support).

To summarise the social support provided and availed of by residents, it was reported by the key workers that over a quarter of

the residents had no family or friends to provide support. For the majority of the residents (62%) it was reported that family and friends were present to provide support, although for 24% doubts as to their ability to provide support was reported. It was reported that 73% of the residents went to visit family and friends and 65% had visits from family and friends. A quarter of the residents reported that they would ask nobody for everyday psychological support or psychological crisis support. The residents reported that they would most likely ask nurses / staff when in need of a small favour, when they wanted to discuss an important decision or when they wanted to talk about something that was upsetting them. In contrast, family and friends were reported as the support network most likely to turn to for everyday psychological support.

6.1.2 *Independence and community integration*

Residents were asked to indicate whether they were aware of the money they received weekly, if they voted and if they left the residences on their own, for example to visit the general practitioner. The majority (71%) of the residents were aware of the amount of money they received each week. Just over half (51%) received help to manage their finances. There were no significant differences in the awareness and management of finances between those in high, medium and low support residences (Chi-square, p > 0.05).

A total of 78% of residents voted. The majority of residents went out on their own (85%). Differences in the proportion of residents from high, medium and low support that reported voting and going out on their own were not statistically significant (Chi-square, p > 0.05). Only 66% of the high support residents visited the GP by themselves, while 84% of the medium support and 84% of low support residents did so.

Residents were asked if they attended particular activities in the community such as bingo, community centres and so on (Table 6.2). Of all residents, only a small percentage reported attending activities in the community with the highest proportion attending pubs etc. (see Table 6.2). There were significant differences in the proportions of residents from high, medium and low support residences attending social clubs (chi-square, p < 0.001), bingo (chi-square, p <

0.01) and community centres (chi-square, p < 0.001). In all cases, a significantly greater proportion of medium support residents attended these activities.

The key workers were asked to rate the residents' motivation in relation to participation in activities taking place in the residences. They reported that 33% of the residents were motivated and actively engaged in activities, 21% wanted to participate but did not have strong motivation to do so and 33% of residents were reported as passively engaging in activities. The key workers reported that 8% of the residents had little understanding of activities and 4% refused to participate.

Only 12% (n = 16) of the residents reported having experienced harassment in the community. Of these, eight had experienced name calling. Four had experienced a random attack in the community (e.g. bag snatched). One participant had experienced sexual harassment and three reported having experienced harassment in psychiatric hospitals they had attended.

6.1.3 Money management

Nursing officers reported that in only 8% of the high support residences were residents unable to look after their own monies. In 92% of the high support residences it was reported by nursing officers that some (81%) or all (11%)

Table 6.2   Number (%) of residents attending activities in the community , by level of support

	High (n = 82)	Medium (n = 25)	Low (n = 31)	Total (n = 138)
Social clubs	4 (4.9)	8 (32.0)	5 (16.1)	17 (12.3)
Bingo	9 (11.0)	6 (24.0)	0	15 (10.9)
Community centres	8 (9.8)	11 (44.0)	2 (6.5)	21 (15.2)
Pubs, clubs, restaurants	37 (45.1)	13 (52.0)	17 (54.8)	67 (48.6)
Leisure centre	5 (6.1)	3 (12.0)	2 (6.5)	10 (7.2)
Library	4 (4.9)	4 (16.0)	3 (9.7)	11 (8.0)
Cinema	24 (29.3)	6 (24.0)	5 (16.1)	53 (25.4)
Religious activities	25 (30.5)	11 (44.0)	7 (22.6)	43 (31.2)

residents were able to look after their own monies, while all the medium and low support residences reported that some (medium 68%, low 41%) or all (medium 32%, low 58%) residents could do so.

6.2 INFORMATION PROVIDED TO RESIDENTS

Questions were asked in the facility questionnaires about the information provided to the residents on rights and complaints procedures, the role and functions of the Mental Health Commission, voting registration and health initiatives. The questionnaire did not address how the information was provided to the residents, however, enquiry was made as to whether notices regarding information on rights and on the complaints procedures were displayed on the walls of the residences. The data concerning the information provided to residents derived from all community residences in the three HSE local areas (n=102) and were provided by the nursing officer in charge of the residences. The nursing officers in the community residences were asked a series of questions relating to the information that was

provided to the residents. The specific questions that were asked are presented in Table 6.3, Table 6.4 and Table 6.5. The tables present the number and the proportion of high, medium and low residences that were reported as providing residents with this information. For completness, the proportion of missing responses (i.e. number of residences that a response was not provided for) is also noted in the table. The analyses below, however, were performed on the completed data and missing categories were excluded.

6.2.1 Information on complaints procedures and rights

Table 6.3 presents the proportion of high, medium and low support residences reporting that information on complaints procedures and rights were provided to residents. In 88% of the residences it was reported that residents were provided with information on rights. The nursing officers were asked if the residents were provided with information on the complaints procedures (i.e. the process of making a complaint within the mental health services)

| Table 6.3 | Information provided to residents on complaints procedures and rights, by level of support |

Information provided		High (n = 36)	Medium (n = 25)	Low (n = 41)
Are residents given information on rights?	Yes	35 (97.2)	21 (84.0)	34 (82.9)
	No	1 (2.8)	3 (12.0)	6 (14.6)
	Missing	0	1 (4.0)	1 (2.5)
	Total	36 (100)	25 (100)	41 (100)
Are residents informed about the complaints procedure?	Yes	33 (91.7)	15 (60.0)	29 (70.7)
	No	3 (8.3)	9 (36.0)	11 (26.8)
	Missing	0	1 (4.0)	1 (2.4)
	Total	36 (100)	25 (100)	41 (100)
Are residents told the name of the local complaints officer?	Yes	27 (75.0)	15 (60.0)	15 (36.6)
	No	8 (22.2)	9 (36.0)	25 (61.0)
	Missing	1 (2.8)	1 (4.0)	1 (2.4)
	Total	36 (100)	25 (100)	41 (100)
Are notices regarding rights and complaints procedures displayed on the walls of the residence?	Yes	19 (52.8)	10 (40.0)	14 (34.1)
	No	17 (47.2)	12 (48.0)	26 (63.4)
	Missing	0	3 (12.0)	1 (2.4)
	Total	36 (100)	25 (100)	41 (100)

Table 6.4   Information provided on the role and functions of the Mental Health Commission, by level of support

	Information Provided	High (n = 36)	Medium (n = 25)	Low (n = 41)
Are residents informed of the Mental Health Commission (role and functions)?	Yes	25 (69.4)	12 (48.0)	14 (34.1)
	No	11 (30.6)	12 (48.0)	25 (61.0)
	Missing	0	1 (4.0)	2 (4.9)

and if they were informed of the name of the local complaints officer. Again, in a large percentage (75%) of the residences it was reported that the residents were provided with information on the complaints procedure. It was reported in a significantly greater proportion of high support residences that the residents received information on complaint procedures (92%) than in the medium (60%) and low (71%) support residences (chi-square, p < 0.05). In contrast, the nursing officers reported that the residents were informed of the name of the local complaints officer in only 54% of the residences. Again, it was reported in a significantly greater proportion of the high support residences (75%) that residents were informed of the name of the complaints officer than in medium (60%) or low (37%) support residences (chi-square, p < 0.01).

Nursing officers were asked whether notices providing residents with information on the complaints procedures and rights were displayed on the walls of the residences. It was reported that this information was displayed on the walls in only 42% of residences. There was no significant difference between the proportions of high, medium or low support facilities reported as displaying this information (Chi-square, p > 0.05). In approximately half of those residences where it was reported that information on rights was provided to the residents, that information was displayed on the walls of the residences. Of those where it was reported that information on the complaints procedures was provided, 54% of the nursing officers reported that the information was on display in the residence.

6.2.2 Information on the Mental Health Commission

It was reported in only half of the residences in the three study areas that residents were provided with information on the roles and functions of the MHC by the staff in the residences. Table 6.4 shows the

Table 6.5   Information provided to residents on voting registration and health initiatives, by level of support

	Information Provided	High (n = 36)	Medium (n = 25)	Low (n = 41)
Are residents asked if they wish to vote and are they assisted in voter registration?	Yes	36 (100)	25 (100)	41 (100)
	No	0	0	0
	Missing	0	0	0
	Total	36 (100)	25 (100)	41 (100)
Are residents informed of national health initiatives (e.g., breast screening) or other health information?	Yes	33 (91.7)	22 (88.0)	37 (90.2)
	No	3 (8.3)	2 (8.0)	4 (9.8)
	Missing	0	1 (4.0)	0
	Total	36 (100)	25 (100)	41 (100)

Table 6.6 *Number of residences (n = 102) providing health information and type of information*

Type of information	Number of residences that provided information
Breast check, smoking cessation	2
Information section on notice board and talks in day centre on a number of health initiatives	1
General health information leaflets from health centers and general practice	7
General health information presented notice boards and in group sessions in the residences	6
Smoking cessation, diet, cancer awareness and educational groups	13
Solutions to wellness programme	6
Talks and literature provided on physical health and mental health	36

proportion of high, medium and low support residences where residents were provided with this information. A total of 69% of nursing officers in the high support residences reported that they informed the residents about the MHC, a significantly greater proportion than that in the medium (48%) or low (34%) support residences (c^2 (4) = 8.64, p < 0.01).

6.2.3 Information on voting registration and health initiatives

Table 6.5 shows the proportion of the residences where it was reported by nursing officers that residents were provided with information on voting registration and that assistance was provided to residents in exercising their voting rights. This is in line with findings in 6.1.2 that 78% of residents reported that they exercised their voting right.

A total of 90% of the residences reported that residents were provided with information on national health initiatives or other health information. The type of health information given, the number of residences providing it and the mode of delivery are presented in Table 6.6.

In 35% of the residences it was reported that residents were

provided with talks and literature on physical and mental health and wellbeing while 13% reported that they specifically provided information on smoking cessation, diet and cancer awareness. Only two nursing officers reported that they specifically provided information on Breast Check. The nursing officers in 14% of the residences reported that they provided general health information in the form of leaflets and talks that were posted on notice boards or delivered within the residences or day centres. In one HSE area (Area B) the residents were given a 'Solutions to Wellness' programme. This was a structured programme that focused on healthy eating and physical exercise.

6.3 SUMMARY

Key workers reported that a quarter of the residents had no family / friends to provide support. The majority of residents' key workers stated that they received visits from relatives and friends and also went out to visit relatives or friends. Regarding the residents' self-reports of social support networks, between 18% and 25% reported that they could not / would not seek support from anyone during times of need. This included everyday psychological support, everyday instrumental support, psychological crisis support or instrumental crisis support. The residents stated that they most often did everyday things with other residents or family and friends from outside the residence. In comparison, support from nurses and care staff was most often sought in times of crisis or decision-making.

The nursing officers reported that in only 8% of the high support residences were none of the residents able to look after their own money, while it was reported that some or all the residents in medium and low support were able to manage their own finances. The majority of residents interviewed indicated that they were aware of how much money they received on a weekly basis, but half received support from the staff to manage their finances.

Most of the residents stated that they went out on their own, that they visited the GP on their own and that they voted. There were no differences in the proportions of high, medium or low support residents that voted, visited the GP by themselves, or went out on their own. Only a small number of residents reported that they attended activities in the community and a greater proportion of the medium and low support residents stated that they did so than the high support residents. The greatest proportion of residents reported that they went to pubs, clubs and restaurants, as opposed to other community activities such as bingo, cinema, social clubs and community centres. Over 10% of the residents had experienced harassment in the community and, in the majority of cases, this had been in the form of name calling.

It was reported by the majority of nursing officers in the residences that residents were provided with information on complaints procedures and rights. However, in just over half of the residences was it stated that residents were provided with the name of the local complaints officer and in less than half that the residence displayed notices about rights and complaints procedures. It was reported in a greater proportion of high support residences that residents were provided with information on rights and complaints procedures. Almost all nursing officers in high support residences stated that they provided such information and three-quarters reported that residents were provided with the name of the local complaints officer.

In few of the residences was it reported that residents were informed about the role and functions of the MHC, although this was more likely to occur in high support residences. This information is especially important for residents who have been or may be involuntarily admitted to psychiatric units or hospitals. This information may be more relevant for this population than for those in medium or low support.

It was indicated in all residences that the residents were provided with support in voting registration. This is congruent with the results from the residents themselves – with nearly 80% reporting that they exercised their voting rights.

Approximately 90% of the nursing officers indicated that information on health initiatives was provided to residents. However few nursing officers reported what these specific health initiatives were when asked to identify what information was provided to residents. The majority of the nursing officers who reported the type of information provided indicated that this concerned general physical and mental health. Smoking cessation, diet and cancer awareness was also provided.

In summary while some information was provided to residents, information on rights and complaints procedures were not made available in all residences nor, more generally, was information on national health initiatives such as cancer screening and prevention and healthy living and diet provided. As reported in Section 4.4.4.5, few residences provided information packs to residents.

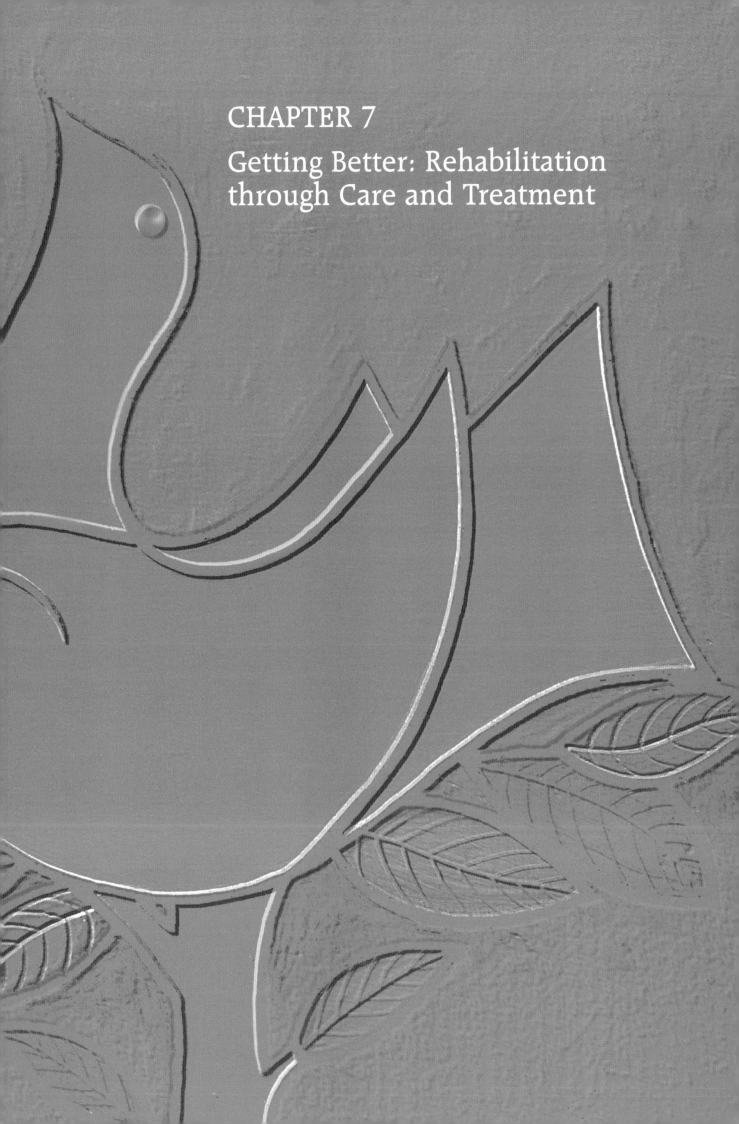

CHAPTER 7
Getting Better: Rehabilitation through Care and Treatment

Chapter 7

Getting better: rehabilitation through care and treatment

This chapter is concerned with the measures taken to reduce the impairments and disabilities of residents by reducing or modifying their level of symptoms and by improving their social functioning.

7.1 SPECIALISED REHABILITATION TEAMS

Two of the three HSE local areas surveyed had specialised rehabilitation teams. Within these two areas there were 29 (9 high support, 13 medium support, 7 low support) community residences reported for the study. All the specialised rehabilitation teams had a consultant psychiatrist, a mental health nurse and social worker. More than two-thirds of the 29 community residences serviced by the specialised rehabilitation teams had an occupational therapist (69%; 20 / 29) and psychologist (65%; 19 / 29) on the multidisciplinary team.

7.2 CARE PRACTICES

Only a small number of residents in medium (8%) and low (29%) support residences were provided with a provisional diagnosis on admission, compared with 58% of high support residents. This is somewhat surprising, given that the majority of the residents would have been well known to the services, but may have resulted from a misunderstanding of the study question (i.e. Is there a provisional admitting diagnosis drawn up once the patient has been admitted?).

7.2.1 *Care plans and key workers*

Nearly all nursing officers in high support residences reported having care plans for residents (97%) as did the medium support residences (92%). The nursing officers in 68% of the low support residences reported having resident care plans. Of those reporting the use of care plans, the majority (96%) reported that the care plans contained information on medical treatment. The nursing officers reported that

only 55% of the residences had care plans that outlined the responsibilities of the team members. They reported that 86% of the residences had care plans that contained documentation indicating diagnosis and 92% had care plans that outlined treatment and rehabilitation activities for the residents.

It was reported that the majority (66%) of the residences had a key worker system in place. A total of 72% of the high support, 84% of the medium support and 49% of the low support residences had a key worker system in place.

7.2.2 *Medication*

Not surprisingly, a total of 98% (n = 135) of the sample of residents were on prescribed medication at the time of the study. Two residents were on no medication and the information was missing for one resident. Table 7.1 shows the number of residents on medication at the time of the study, by level of support. Totals in the table refer to multiple responses (i.e. an individual could be in more than one category) and therefore, totals for high, medium and low support do not match sample totals. The totals presented in the table are the row percentages. Of the residents on medication at the time of the study (n = 135), the majority of residents (85%) were on Clozapine or other atypical antipsychotic medication. A total of 49% of residents were on typical antipsychotic drugs. Key workers reported that 16 residents were prescribed atypical and typical antipsychotic drugs simultaneously at the time of the study. A total of eight residents were prescribed both Clozapine and another atypical antipsychotic drug at the time of the study. There was no overlap between Clozapine and typical antipsychotic drugs (i.e. no resident was prescribed Clozapine and a typical antipsychotic drug).

Table 7.1   Number (%) of residents on medication, by category, by level of support

Medication	High	Medium	Low	Total
Clozapine and other atypical antipsychotic drug	71 (61.7)	16 (13.9)	28 (24.3)	115 (100)
Typical antipsychotic drug	49 (74.2)	9 (13.6)	8 (12.1)	66 (100)
Antidepressant	21 (58.3)	9 (25.0)	6 (16.7)	36 (100)
Bipolar disorder drug	27 (77.1)	4 (11.4)	4 (11.4)	35 (100)
Other psychotropic drug	18 (81.8)	0	4 (18.2)	22 (100)
Anti-Parksonian drug	27 (64.3)	10 (23.8)	5 (11.9)	42 (100)
Hypnotic	21 (67.7)	6 (19.4)	4 (12.9)	31 (100)
Total	234 (67.5%)	54 (15.5%)	59 (17.0%)	347 (100%)

A total of 86% (71 / 82) of high support residents were prescribed atypical antipsychotic drugs, while 60% (49 / 82) were prescribed typical antipsychotic drugs. Of the medium support residents, 64% (16 / 25) were prescribed antipsychotic drugs, with 36% (9 / 25) on typical antipsychotic drugs. The corresponding proportions for low support residents were 90% (28 / 31) for atypical antipsychotic drugs and 26% (8 / 31) for typical antipsychotic drugs. In addition, a total of 26% (21 / 82) of high support, 36% (9 / 25) of medium support and 19% (6 / 31) of low support residents were on antidepressants at the time of the study. There was a greater proportion of medium support residents (36%; 4 / 25) on bipolar disorder drugs than high (26%; 27 / 82) or low (19%; 4 / 31) support residents. This pattern was the same for anti-Parkinsonian drugs (medium 40%; high 33%; low 16%). Finally, the proportion of high support residents on hypnotics (26%; 21 / 82) was similar to the proportion of medium support residents (24%; 6 / 25); while a lower proportion of low support residents were on hypnotics (13%; 4 / 31).

7.3   ATTENDANCE AT DAY CENTRES / DAY HOSPITALS

This section refers to the total number of residents (n = 871) in the three areas across all 102 facilities. It was reported by nursing officers that 40% (349 / 871) of residents attended a day centre or day hospital. Of these, 30% (168 / 554) were high support residents, 57% (88 / 153) were medium support residents and 57% (93 / 164) were low support residents. Table 7.2 shows the number of residences reporting the proportion of residents that were attending day centres or day hospitals. Analysis revealed that only 17% of the high support residences had 81% to 100% of residents attending day residences, compared to 24% of the medium support residences and nearly half (46%) of the low support residences. A quarter of the high support residences had no residents attending day centres or day hospitals, compared to 8% of the medium and 22% of the low support residences.

7.4   REHABILITATIVE TRAINING AND ACTIVITIES TO PROMOTE WELLBEING

Table 7.3 shows the activities provided for residents. In nearly all cases, a greater proportion of the high support residences than the lower support residences provided activities for the residents. However, less than half of the high support residences provided vocational training (44%) compared to 60% of the medium support and 39% of the low

Table 7.2   Number (%) of residences showing the proportion of residents attending either day centres or day hospitals, by level of support

% of residents attending	High (n = 36)	Medium (n = 25)	Low (n = 41)	Total (n = 102)
None	9 (25.0)	2 (8.0)	9 (22.0)	20 (19.6)
1% – 20%	10 (27.8)	1 (4.0)	1 (2.4)	12 (11.8)
21% – 40%	7 (19.4)	6 (24.0)	6 (14.6)	19 (18.6)
41% – 60%	2 (5.6)	6 (24.0)	2 (4.9)	10 (9.8)
61% – 80%	2 (5.6)	4 (16.0)	4 (9.8)	10 (9.8)
81% – 100%	6 (16.7)	6 (24.0)	19 (46.3)	31 (30.4)

support residences. Very few of the residences provided cognitive behavioural therapy (high support 22%, medium support 16% and low support 12%). The majority of high, medium and low support provided practical living skills, social skills training and budget training. Nearly all the high support (94%) and a smaller proportion of medium (68%) and low (61%) support residences provided leisure activities. It was reported by the nursing officers that fewer than one-third of the residences provided family education programmes (31%). Of the high support residences, 44% provided such programmes, while only 28% of the medium and 22% of low support residences did so.

7.5 COMMUNITY INTEGRATION

Table 7.4 shows activities that were provided to aid community integration and the proportion of residences providing these activities. A large proportion of the residences provided activities to promote community integration (67%). A total of 52% of the residences provided activities that involved members of the local community and 63% participated in events organised by community groups with a greater proportion of high support facilities providing these activities. It was reported in less than half of the high support residences that activities to encourage work (39%) or collaboration with others to find employment for

Table 7.3   Number (%) of residences providing activities and training, by level of support

	High (n = 36)	Medium (n = 25)	Low (n = 41)	Total (n = 102)
Vocational training	16 (44.4)	15 (60.0)	16 (39.0)	47 (46.1)
Cognitive behavioural therapy	8 (22.2)	4 (16.0)	5 (12.2)	17 (16.7)
Practical living skills	34 (94.4)	19 (76.0)	34 (82.9)	87 (85.3)
Social skills training	32 (88.9)	18 (72.0)	29 (70.7)	79 (77.5)
Budget training	29 (80.6)	16 (64.0)	26 (63.4)	71 (69.6)
Physical activities	31 (86.1)	11 (44.0)	21 (51.2)	63 (61.8)
Addiction counselling	11 (30.6)	5 (20.0)	11 (26.8)	27 (26.5)
Family education	16 (44.4)	7 (28.0)	9 (22.0)	32 (31.4)
Leisure activities	34 (94.4)	17 (68.0)	25 (61.0)	76 (74.5)

Table 7.4	Number (%) of residences providing activities to aid community integration, by level of support			
	High (n = 36)	Medium (n = 25)	Low (n = 41)	Total (n = 102)
Activities to involve community members	23 (63.8)	10 (40.0)	20 (48.8)	53 (52.0)
Activities to promote community integration	27 (75.0)	16 (64.0)	25 (61.0)	68 (66.6)
Activities to encourage work	13 (36.1)	7 (29.2)	20 (51.3)	40 (39.2)
Events organised by community groups	25 (69.4)	15 (60.0)	24 (58.5)	64 (62.7)
Collaboration with others to find employment	13 (36.1)	10 (41.7)	21 (53.8)	44 (43.1)
Activities to facilitate rehousing	19 (52.7)	10 (40.0)	27 (67.5)	56 (54.9)

residents (43%) was provided. Just over half of the high support residences encouraged rehousing (55%), with 40% of the medium support and 67% of the low support residences doing so.

7.6 INDEPENDENT AND ORGANISED HOLIDAYS

The nursing officers in the residences were asked to indicate the number of residents that had been on independent or organised holidays in the last two years. Independent holidays referred to holidays that were organised by the resident themselves. Organised holidays referred to holidays organised by the staff of the residences. Table 7.5 and Table 7.6 show the proportion of residents who went on independent or organised holidays in the last two years.

A total of 19% (n = 168) of residents were reported to have gone on independent holidays in the last two years, while just less than half (44%; n = 385) went on organised holidays. A total of 13% of high support residents went on independent holidays, while less than one third of medium support residents and 27% of low support residents went on independent holidays). Regarding organised holidays, 41% of the high support residents, 46% of medium support residents and 54% of the low support residents opted to go on these holidays in the last two years. A third of the residences (33%) reported that none of the residents went on independent holidays over the last two years (Table 7.5),

Table 7.5	Number (%) of residences showing the proportion of residents going on independent holidays in the past two years, by level of support			
% of residents	High (n = 36)	Medium (n = 25)	Low (n = 41)	Total (n = 102)
None	10 (27.8)	9 (36.0)	15 (36.6)	34 (33.3)
1% –20%	17 (47.2)	2 (8.0)	4 (9.8)	23 (22.5)
21% – 40%	8 (22.2)	6 (24.0)	12 (29.3)	26 (25.5)
41% – 60%	1 (2.8)	4 (16.0)	5 (12.2)	10 (9.8)
61% – 80%	0	1 (4.0)	4 (9.8)	5 (4.9)
81% – 100%	0	3 (2.9)	1 (2.4)	4 (3.9)

Table 7.6   Number (%) of residences showing the proportion of residents going on organised holidays in the last two years, by level of support

% of residents	High (n = 36)	Medium (n = 25)	Low (n = 41)	Total (n = 102)
None	9 (25.0)	6 (24.0)	6 (14.6)	21 (20.6)
1% –20%	5 (13.9)	1 (4.0)	2 (4.9)	8 (7.8)
21% – 40%	4 (11.1)	4 (11.1)	8 (19.5)	16 (15.7)
41% – 60%	5 (13.9)	7 (28.0)	5 (12.2)	17 (16.7)
61% – 80%	3 (8.3)	2 (8.0)	9 (22.0)	14 (13.7)
81% – 100%	10 (27.8)	5 (20.0)	11 (26.8)	26 (25.5)

while 21% reported that none of the residents went on organised holidays (Table 7.6).

7.7   SUMMARY

Two of the HSE local areas had consultant-led specialist rehabilitation teams. More high support (58%) than medium (8%) and low support residences (29%) were provided with provisional diagnoses of residents on their admission. The great majority of high and medium support residences reported having care plans for residents, as compared to 68% of low support residences. Ninety-eight per cent of residents were on prescribed medication at the time of the study. No less than 85% of residents were on Clozapine or other atypical anti-psychotics and 49% of the 135 residents on medication were on typical anti-psychotics with 16 residents taking both atypicals and typicals simultaneously; however, no resident was taking Clozapine and a typical anti-psychotic at the same time. The highest proportions of residents on anti-psychotics, atypical and typical, were those in high support. Just over a quarter of residents were prescribed anti-depressants. In addition, a sizeable proportion of residents were taking medication for bipolar disorder, medication to counter side effects of anti-psychotics, hypnotics or other medications.

A greater proportion of high support than of lower support residences provided activities of a rehabilitative or training nature. Only 44% of high support residences, compared to 60% of medium support residences, made vocational training available and cognitive behavioural therapy was provided in less than one-fifth of residences. However, training in practical living skills and social training and instruction in budgeting were undertaken in the majority of residences. Physical and leisure-time activities were the rule in most residences. A range of other activities was undertaken in many residences.

Efforts to encourage community integration were in progress in over two-thirds of residences – more so in high support than in medium and low support settings. On the other hand less than half of residences undertook initiatives to help residents find employment, whereas matters were somewhat better in relation to having residents seek rehousing.

The results showed that a greater proportion of residents in medium and low support than in high support residences went on holidays, either independently or organised by the services. A very small proportion of residents from high support went on independent holidays while a greater proportion went on supervised holidays. Overall, only a small proportion of residents had been on holiday in the last two years, either on their own or with the staff from the residences. .

CHAPTER 8

Our View: Residents'
Satisfaction with Care and
Treatment and Other Aspects
of Life

Chapter 8

Our view: residents' satisfaction with care and treatment and other aspects of life

All the information reported in this chapter concerns the residents' views of their lives in the community residential facilities.

8.1 SATISFACTION WITH, AND PREFERENCE FOR, ACCOMMODATION

The residents were asked if they wished to stay in their current accommodation and if they had a choice where they would prefer to live. A total of 76% (n = 105) of the residents were willing to stay in their current accommodation. The residents in medium support facilities appeared most content with their accommodation, in that 96% indicated a willingness to remain in their community homes compared to only 68% of the high support and 81% of the low support residents. A large proportion of the residents (59%; n = 82) were happy where they were (high support 52%; medium support 80%; low support 61%). Of those who, if given the choice, would like to move (n = 56), the majority would prefer independent living (20%; n = 28) or to live at home (13%; n = 18). A total of 40% of the high support residents would prefer independent living or would prefer to live at home. By comparison, 16% of the medium support and 29% of the low support residents would prefer independent living or living at home. Only 7.2% residents reported that they would prefer to live in a group home or another hostel.

8.2 RESIDENTS' SATISFACTION WITH TREATMENT AND CARE

Table 8.1 presents the questions that residents were asked regarding their care plans. Totals refer to the number of residents who responded to the questions.

Only 20% of the residents reported that they had knowledge of their care plans. For those who reported that they were unsure or did not know, the researcher explained the term care plan so that the remaining questions could be asked. Of all residents, 21% reported that they were involved in drawing up their care plan; 24% reported that their care plan had been explained to them prior to the interview; 27% reported that they knew when their care plan would be reviewed. Nearly two-thirds of the residents (64%) reported that they knew what their medication was for, and 46% reported that they knew about the possible side effects of their medication.

Residents were also asked a number of questions regarding their satisfaction with their key worker (see Table 8.2). Just over a quarter (29%) of the residents reported that the term key worker had been explained to them. For those who reported that they were unsure or did not know, the researcher explained the term key worker so that the remaining questions could be asked. It appeared to the researcher on a number of occasions that the residents in high support residences were answering the questions in relation

Table 8.1	Residents' responses to statements about their care plans (number and percentages)			
	Yes	Not sure	No	Total
I know what my care plan is.	27 *(20)*	17 *(12)*	92 *(68)*	136 *(100)*
I was involved in drawing up my care plan.	29 *(21)*	21 *(15)*	86 *(63)*	136 *(100)*
My care plan has been explained to me.	33 *(24)*	20 *(15)*	83 *(61)*	136 *(100)*
I know what my medication is for.	86 *(64)*	30 *(22)*	19 *(14)*	135 *(100)*
I know the possible side effects of my medication.	62 *(46)*	24 *(17)*	49 *(36)*	135 *(100)*
I know when my care plan is going to be reviewed.	37 *(27)*	41 *(30)*	58 *(43)*	136 *(100)*

Table 8.2   Residents' responses to statements about treatment and care provided by key workers (numbers and percentages)

	Yes	Not sure	No	Total
The term key worker has been explained to me.	39 (29.3)	12 (9.0)	82 (61.6)	133 (100.0)
I know the name of my key worker.	70 (52.6)	17 (12.8)	46 (34.6)	133 (100.0)
My key worker has explained to me their view of my problems.	75 (56.4)	19 (14.3)	39 (29.3)	133 (100.0)
My key worker is helping me cope with my mental health problems.	96 (72.2)	17 (12.8)	20 (15.0)	133 (100.0)
If I have a problem I can easily contact my key worker.	99 (74.4)	16 (12.0)	18 (13.5)	133 (100.0)
My key worker helps me with practical problems.	96 (72.2)	16 (12.0)	21 (15.8)	133 (100.0)
I can easily talk about my personal problems with my key worker.	90 (67.7)	19 (14.3)	24 (18.0)	133 (100.0)
My key worker lets my GP know how I am getting on.	79 (59.4)	23 (17.3)	31 (23.3)	133 (100.0)
I can always rely on my key worker to show up at arranged times.	87 (65.4)	25 (18.8)	21 (15.8)	133 (100.0)
My key worker helps make sure I keep my appointment with the psychiatrist.	78 (58.6)	27 (20.3)	28 (21.0)	133 (100.0)
My key worker makes sure I am all right if I don't turn up for an appointment.	77 (57.9)	30 (22.5)	26 (19.6)	133 (100.0)

to the nurse in charge of the residence, as they appeared not to have a specific key worker assigned to them. Less than half of the high support residents (43%) reported that they knew the name of their key worker. The majority (67%) of the high support residents, however, stated that the nurses who worked in the residence provided them with practical help. While residents may not have had or were unaware of the identity of their key worker, a large percentage reported that they were getting support from nurses.

Of the total sample of residents, just over half (53%) said they knew the name of their key worker and 56% reported that the key worker had explained to them their view of their problems. Nearly two-thirds (72%) felt that their key worker was helping them to cope and 74% indicated that their key worker was easy to contact, when necessary. Regarding help with problems, again nearly two-thirds (72%) felt that the key worker helped them with

practical problems and 68% felt they could easily talk to their key worker about personal problems. Fifty-nine percent of the residents reported that the key worker kept the GP informed of their progress and also made sure that they kept their appointments with the psychiatrist. A large proportion of the residents indicated that they could rely on the key worker to turn up at arranged times (65%) and 58% reported that the key worker would check that they were all right if they missed an appointment.

Regarding support from the psychiatrist, over half of the residents (63%) felt that they could easily talk to their psychiatrist about personal problems and 71% felt that the psychiatrist was helping them with their mental health problems. Only half (51%) of the residents reported that the psychiatrist explained their problems to them. Likewise, just over half (57%) felt that the psychiatrist kept them informed of their progress, with 43% reporting that the psychiatrist explained how their problems affected their lives.

The majority of residents stated that they were 'quite happy' or 'very happy' with the treatment and care provided (85%). Only 12% reported that they were 'not very happy' or 'not at all happy'. A total of 63% of the sample reported that they had 'enough information' on their illness. Only 10% reported that they had received 'no information' or 'little information' on their illness. A total of 24% stated that they would have liked more information on their mental health problems.

8.3 RESIDENTS' SELF-REPORTED QUALITY OF LIFE AND PERCEPTIONS OF LIFE IN THE RESIDENCE

Residents were asked to rate their quality of life on 18 items. The items were scored on a three-point scale from 0 – 2, with higher scores indicating greater satisfaction. The scores on the 18 items were summed to give a total quality of life score. Total scores could range from 0 to 36. There was a significant difference between the levels of support on the Quality of Life Questionnaire (F (Kruskal Wallis Test, $p < 0.01$). Residents from high support residences reported significantly lower quality of life (30.0; range 0 – 41) than residents from medium (33.7; range 21 – 36) or low (33.1; range 21 – 42) support residences.

Residents were asked to rate their perceptions of life in the residence on 12 items. The items were scored on a four-point scale from 0 – 3, with higher scores indicating more positive perceptions. There were no significant differences between level of support on the twelve individual items ($p > 0.05$). The residents' perceptions of life in the residences were mostly positive. A total of 67% of the residents reported that they thought it was 'good' or 'great' to live in their current accommodation and a similar proportion (66%) felt that the atmosphere within the residence was positive most or all of the time. The majority of the residents

indicated that residents got on well together (75%) and felt that the staff got on well with residents (81%). Regarding activities during the day, only 6% reported that they were bored during the weekdays 'all of the time' or 'most of the time', while 8% felt bored 'all of the time' or 'most of the time' at weekends. Just over a third (39%) of residents felt that they had a 'moderate' or 'a lot' of say in the day-to-day running of the household; however, almost two-thirds (72%) reported that they were 'happy most of the time' or 'very happy' with their involvement in the running of the residence. Likewise, over half the residents reported that they had 'no input' or 'little input' with regard to their treatment (55%). Only a small proportion of residents felt that they had 'no control' or 'little' control over how they lead their lives (7.8%), with over two-thirds reporting 'moderate' to 'a lot' of control (76%). In addition, the majority of residents were 'happy most of the time' or 'very happy' with their level of independence (75%) and were happy with their involvement in the community (76%).

8.4 QUALITATIVE ANALYSIS OF RESIDENTS' COMMENTS

Of the 138 participants in the study sample, 90% (n = 124) provided responses to open-ended questions. The residents were asked to tell the interviewer 'a bit about what it was like to live here in their current accommodation'. The following prompts were used to guide the conversation:

☐ What are the best bits about living here?

☐ What are the worst bits?

☐ What would you improve?

☐ Where do you see yourself living in the future?

☐ What are your hopes for the future?

The information provided by the residents was analysed using SPSS for Text Analysis. A total of eight main categories were

Table 8.3   Total number (%) of residents providing comments under the main themes, by level of support (n = 124)

Main themes		Level of support			
		High	Medium	Low	Total
Accommodation	Happy here	44 *(54.3)*	17 *(21.0)*	20 *(24.7)*	81 *(100.0)*
	Independent living	17 *(58.6)*	2 *(6.9)*	10 *(34.5)*	29 *(100.0)*
	Would like to go home	16 *(84.2)*	1 *(5.3)*	2 *(10.5)*	19 *(100.0)*
	Perceive residence as home	1 *(33.3)*	1 *(33.3)*	1 *(33.3)*	3 *(100.0)*
	Own room	10 *(52.6)*	3 *(15.8)*	6 *(31.6)*	19 *(100.0)*
	Sharing room	3 *(75.0)*		1 *(25.0)*	4 *(100.0)*
Food	Food - positive	10 *(71.4)*	1 *(7.1)*	3 *(21.4)*	14 *(100.0)*
	Food - negative	6 *(66.7)*	2 *(22.2)*	1 *(11.1)*	9 *(100.0)*
Residents	Residents - positive	7 *(58.3)*	3 *(25.0)*	2 *(16.7)*	12 *(100.0)*
	Residents - negative	9 *(69.2)*	2 *(15.4)*	2 *(15.4)*	13 *(100.0)*
Nursing and staff	Nurses and staff - negative	7 *(50.0)*	1 *(7.1)*	6 *(42.9)*	14 *(100.0)*
	Nurses and staff - positive	15 *(60.0)*	4 *(16.0)*	6 *(24.0)*	25 *(100.0)*
Doctor	Doctor - positive	1 *(50.0)*	1 *(50.0)*		2 *(100.0)*
	Doctor - negative	8 *(80.0)*	1 *(10.0)*	1 *(10.0)*	10 *(100.0)*
Medication	Medication - negative	8 *(53.3)*	1 *(6.7)*	6 *(40.0)*	15 *(100.0)*
	Medication - positive	3 *(75.0)*	1 *(25.0)*		4 *(100.0)*
Finances	Money - negative	10 *(90.9)*	1 *(9.1)*		11 *(100.0)*
	Money - positive	2 *(66.7)*		1 *(33.3)*	3 *(100.0)*
Employment	Would like to work	9 *(56.3)*	3 *(18.8)*	4 *(25.0)*	16 *(100.0)*
Future	Hopes for future – negative	11 *(68.8)*	2 *(12.5)*	3 *(18.8)*	16 *(100.0)*
	Hopes for future - positive	17 *(58.6)*	3 *(10.3)*	9 *(31.0)*	29 *(100.0)*
	Total	73 *(58.9)*	22 *(17.7)*	29 *(23.4)*	124 *(100.0)*

extracted during data analysis. These categories included accommodation, other residents, nurses and staff, psychiatrists and doctors, medication, finances, hopes for the future and work. The categories included both negative and positive responses. The frequency of responses and examples of the residents' views taken from researchers' notes are presented below. Table 8.3 shows the frequencies of the positive and negative responses within these categories from high, medium and low residents.

8.4.1 Accommodation

Responses in this category included the residents' satisfaction with current accommodation, preference for accommodation, room sharing and food. A total of 81 (65%) of respondents reported that they were happy in their current accommodation, at least for the present.

☐ Comfortable and good food. Nurse will go shopping with you

However, nearly a quarter of the respondents indicated that they would like to move, either now or eventually, to independent living – an apartment of their own (23%) and 19 (15%) reported that they would like to go back to their own home. Some residents acknowledged the benefit of the current accommodation and the supports provided, but stated that they would like to move in the future. Other residents recognised the need for support even if they were living independently. It is interesting to note that only three respondents referred to the residence as home.

☐ *Would like to go home in the future with some support.*

☐ *Group home is grand. Eventually would like my own place. Name on waiting list, but about six year wait.*

☐ *So happy here – staff are excellent. In the future would like to go home and get part-time job and eventually a council flat.*

Only four (3%) residents reported that they liked sharing a room. The comments made by these residents suggested that they liked having the company and had shared a room for so long that they would be lonely if in a room by themselves. On the other hand, more residents raised the issue of single rooms (15%, n = 15). For those who had their own rooms, they stated that the privacy of single rooms was a great benefit when sharing accommodation. Likewise, residents who were sharing rooms, felt that single rooms would offer more privacy.

☐ *Better than the streets but overcrowded, no privacy.*

☐ *Good that I can have visitors. Have my own room.*

☐ *Would like more privacy, but no man is an island, you have to depend on others.*

Food in the residence was referred to by 18% of the respondents, with 14 (61%) making positive comments about the food and 9 (39%) making negative comments. Positive comments mainly referred to good food. The negative food comments in general referred to the fact that residents did not have a choice in the type of food they ate or in fact, when they ate it. In addition, the lack of kitchen facilities to cook your own food was highlighted.

☐ *Food is good. Share a room – don't mind.*

☐ *Not good that you can't make your own tea. Can't choose what to eat.*

☐ *Food could be better.*

8.4.2 Residents

This category referred to comments made regarding the other residents in the residence. There were 25 responses in this category. Of these, 48% (12) were positive comments, while 52% (13) were negative comments. The positive comments referred to the fact that residents got on well together as did residents and nursing staff. However, it was also pointed out there were too many people in some residences and that it was difficult to live with people 24 hours per day when you don't get along with them.

☐ *Difficult to deal with other people.*

☐ *Happy to stay here, but do not like one woman. Blames you for everything.*

☐ *Great friends with others.*

☐ *Too many people here.*

8.4.3 Nurses and staff

A total of 14 (11%) residents made negative comments about the staff (nurses, care workers). These residents most often commented that the nursing staff did not take their views into account regarding medication, health and well-being and their willingness to go home.

☐ *District nurse wouldn't let me go home. Can't take it anymore – not being able to go home. I'm better now – no illness, should be able to go home. Nurses won't let me.*

☐ *Need to build a relationship with nurses. They are a bit bossy.*

Notwithstanding this, a greater proportion (20%, n = 25) of the residents made positive comments about the staff referring to their understanding and support they provided to the residents.

- ☐ *Staff are nice and look after people well.*

- ☐ *Staff are very good, nice and helpful.*

- ☐ *Supervisor is very good, arranges everything for you, they do your chores.*

- ☐ *Good supervisors and great to have support.*

8.4.4 Psychiatrists and doctors

Interestingly only two positive comments were made about the doctors while ten negative comments were made. These generally made reference to the lack of consultations with the doctor and frequent change in doctors.

"Would like to see the psychiatrist more often."

"Psychiatrist change very often, cannot easily talk to them."

"I see a psychiatrist every six weeks, which is not helpful."

8.4.5 Medication

There were 19 comments regarding medication. Of these, four positive comments (21%) were made about the effects of the medication while 15 (79%) comments were made regarding the negative effects of medication. These comments highlighted that residents wanted to have input into their medication, but were often not listened too.

"I would like more rehabilitation. Feel disoriented after ECT."

"Asked the doctor to get medication changed and they said this was the best medication."

"Get injections once a month and I don't need it. Would like to get it twice a year."

"Would like to know more about medication and have it reduced."

"The worst is that you cannot self-medicate."

8.4.6 Finance

A total of 14 (11%) people raised the topic of finance and a large proportion voiced thier concerns about money (78%). Residents were concerned that they were not managing their own money and were only given a certain amount to live on each week. They felt that the allocated amount was not enough and that they should be allowed to spend it as they want.

"Did not have enough money to buy cigarettes. Had to quit smoking."

"Should let me go to the pub. What happens to the rest of the money after cigarettes? Why save when you are 74, only to leave it behind. I want the 54 Euro that I have left. Don't want to save it."

"I am worried that someone will take my money from the bank if I have too much."

"Don't know where my money is."

"Out of 160 Euro I get just 40. I was paying rent of 70 Euro and now I am not. I am a bit traumatised by that."

8.4.7 Hopes for the future

There was a total of 45 comments made regarding hope for the future. Of these, 16 comments (35%) indicated that residents had no hopes for the future or didn't think about the future. A total of 29 comments (64%) were made regarding positive hopes for the future. These hopes generally referred to the residents getting their own accommodation and entering the work force.

"In the future I would like a simple job and more money for a house."

"In the future I would like to go to another place or flats in another place."

"I would like to leave here and get better. Doctor told me it will be 2

– 5 years before I get home."

"My hopes are that I complete my course by Christmas and that I manage my health to a level that I don't have to go to hospital."

"Future – haven't thought about it."

"Happy living here. Not thinking about the future, take one day at a time."

8.4.8 Work

A total of 16 comments (13%) were made regarding work. The majority of these were made in relation to hopes for getting work in the future.

"Future – would like to go to a group home and after a while get part-time work / community scheme."

"Hope to get another job and place to live on my own."

"Waiting on community employment scheme. Waiting for six months."

"Would like to get back to work."

8.5   SUMMARY

The majority of the residents reported that they wanted to stay in their current accommodation. The analysis of responses to the open ended questions qualifies these results to some extent. The residents felt that the current accommodation was comfortable and positive comments were made regarding the quality of the food. A substantial number of the residents, however, reported that, if they had a choice, they would prefer to be at home or in accommodation of their own.

Generally, the residents reported that they were satisfied with their treatment and care. While few residents knew what their care plan was, when it was explained, they reported that they had one somewhere. The majority reported that they knew what their medication was for. The qualitative results suggested that the residents had a negative view of the medication, and this was in terms of not having control over the medication that they were taking. A number of residents reported that they had asked questions regarding changing the medication with the medical staff, but they felt that they were not listened to. Just over a quarter of the residents reported that they had the term key worker explained to them. When the researcher explained the term key worker, over half of the residents reported that they knew the name of their key worker. Overall, the majority of residents were satisfied with the treatment and care provided by the key worker, or where there was not a key worker, by the nurses or care staff in the residences. The majority of the residents reported that the key worker helped them with practical problems and that they could easily talk to their key worker about personal problems. This corresponds to self-reports of the social support network, where the majority of residents reported that they would ask staff for help with small favours and with crises (Section 6.1.1). The majority of residents also reported that they could talk easily to the psychiatrist and that he / she was helping them to cope. However, comments from the residents suggested that the psychiatrists changed too often and that they did not attend the psychiatrist as often as they would like. Generally the residents reported that they were happy with the treatment and care they received. A quarter of the residents reported that they would like more information on their problems; while the majority reported that they had enough information.

Overall, the residents had high scores on the quality of life questionnaire suggesting that they were satisfied with most areas of their lives. The residents in the medium and low support residences were significantly more satisfied than those in high support. The residents' comments suggested that they had hopes for the future, and these hopes were: to get better, get their own accommodation and improve their occupational functioning.

The residents' perceptions of life in the residences were mostly positive. This was evident in the comments made by the residents especially in terms of relationships between residents and between residents and staff. They also reported that the atmosphere in the residence was generally good. Some residents, however, made comments regarding the lack of privacy and not having access to single rooms. Few residents reported that they were bored during the weekdays, with slightly more reporting boredom during the weekends. The results showed that residents had little input to the running of the residences, but the majority were happy with this situation. The majority of the residents reported that they could lead their life as they wanted and that they were happy with their current level of independence. It must be noted that, while residents reported being happy with their level of independence on the questionnaire, their comments indicted that they hoped to improve their current situation and this most often included gaining greater independence from the services. The residents' responses to the questionnaires were qualified and elaborated on in response to the open-ended questions. This issue is further addressed in Chapter 10.

CHAPTER 9
Our Roles: Staff Views of Community Residences

Chapter 9

Our roles: staff views of community residences

This chapter describes the staffing of community residences, staff perceptions of the role and function of residences and the factors that promoted or constrained independence and progression to independent community living.

9.1   STAFFING LEVELS WITHIN THE COMMUNITY RESIDENCES

Nursing officers from participating high support residences reported the number of staff including nursing staff, care staff and household staff working at three time-intervals throughout the day (morning shift 8am to 2pm, afternoon shift 2pm to 8pm and night shift 8pm to 8am). Staffing levels within this shift rota were reported for the majority of residences; however, some residences had slightly different rotas. Some residences had staff employed on a part time basis, thus it was possible for residences to have 0.5 staff on a given shift. As expected, the low support residences had no staff present on a full-time basis, but had regular visits from nursing staff. The medium support residences had night-time supervision by non-nursing staff. These residences had, on average, one care staff on the night

shift and few had staff during the morning or afternoon shift.

There was an average of 2.37 and 2.25 nursing staff in the high support residences in the morning and afternoon shifts, respectively. There were slightly fewer nurses on the night shift (mean 1.72). The average number of care staff was 0.25 for the morning and the afternoon shifts and the average number of household staff for these shifts was 1.15 and 1.05. The average number of staff in the high support residences was calculated for a 24-hour period. During a 24 hour period there was on average 6.34 nurses, 0.50 care staff and 2.15 household staff. This resulted in an estimated total average staff number of 8.99 staff working in the high support residences within a 24-hour period.

Table 9.1 shows the number of high support residences within each staffing level category at each shift. The majority of the high support residences had less than three nurses on duty during the morning (83%), afternoon (86%) and night shift (94%). Regarding household staff, the high support residences had approximately

Table 9.1	Number (%) of high support residences within each staffing level, by shift		
	Morning	Afternoon	Night
1 - 2.9 nurses	30 (83.3)	31 (86.1)	34 (94.4)
1 - 2.9 care staff	8 (22.2)	8 (22.2)	13 (36.1)
1 - 2.9 household staff	27 (75.0)	23 (63.8)	0
3 – 4.9 nurses	4 (11.1)	3 (8.3)	2 (5.5)
3 – 4.9 care staff	0	0	0
3 – 4.9 household staff	1 (2.7)	1 (2.7)	0
5 – 6.9 nurses	1 (2.7)	1 (2.7)	0
5 – 6.9 care staff	0	0	0
5 – 6.9 household staff	0	0	0
7 – 8.9 nurses	1 (2.7)	1 (2.7)	0
7 – 8.9 care staff	0	0	0
7 – 8.9 household staff	0	0	0

Table 9.2   Number (%) of staff, by occupation, by level of support

Occupation	High	Medium	Low	Total
Mental health nurse	29 (85.5)	3 (30.0)	7 (87.5)	39 (75.0)
Care worker	1 (2.9)	6 (60.0)	1 (12.5)	8 (15.4)
Care assistant	0	1 (10.0)	0	1 (1.9)
Domestic staff	2 (5.9)	0	0	2 (3.8)
Other	2 (5.9)	0	0	2 (3.8)
Total	34 (100)	10 (100)	8 (100)	52 (100)

one household staff and one care staff for the morning and afternoon shifts.

The nursing officers reported that a total of 26% (n = 27) of the residences had trainees or volunteers on placement. Of the high support residences, 79% had trainees or volunteers within the residences. A total of 7% of the medium support and 15% of the low support residences had trainees / volunteers on placement.

The majority of the medium and low support residences had emergency staff on call on weekdays (medium 88%; low 61%). Few had emergency staff on call on Saturdays (medium 24%; low 36%), on Sundays or public holidays (medium 24%; low 36%).

9.2   STAFF PERCEPTIONS OF THE AIMS AND FUNCTIONS OF COMMUNITY RESIDENCES

Information is now presented on staff perceptions of the aims and functions of community residences. The staff on duty in the residences where the sample of residents was interviewed were asked to participate . No staff member refused to participate. The majority of staff completed the questionnaire and returned it to the researchers while they were on site. The questionnaires provided staff with a list of eight functions of the community residences and staff members were required to rate these functions on level of importance (see Appendix 4 for questionnaire). The questionnaire also

Table 9.3   Number (%) of staff rating the importance of the aims and functions

Aims and functions	No importance	Moderate importance	High importance	Question unanswered
Service to shorten inpatient treatment	11 (21.2)	8 (15.4)	28 (53.8)	5 (9.6)
Alternative to inpatient care	12 (23.1)	9 (17.3)	27 (51.9)	4 (7.7)
Failure of outpatient care/ day care/ home care	13 (25.0)	12 (23.1)	21 (40.4)	6 (11.5)
Crisis intervention	15 (28.8)	10 (19.2)	23 (44.2)	4 (7.7)
Rehabilitation to independent living / lower support	2 (3.9)	1 (2.0)	47 (90.4)	2 (3.8)
Psychosocial rehabilitation and support	0	1 (2.0)	49 (94.2)	2 (3.8)
Home for life	6 (11.5)	6 (11.5)	40 (77.0)	0
Respite care	14 (26.9)	8 (15.4)	26 (50.0)	4 (7.7)

Table 9.4   Number (%) of responses in each category of factors believed to promote independent living

Categories	N = 126(%)
Support from staff team – well trained, encouraging, trust, respect, good environment/atmosphere	27 (21.4)
Independence/responsibility/making decisions/choice/participation	26 (20.6)
Community support and community involvement	21 (16.7)
Training/education/guidance/rehabilitation	18 (14.3)
Confidence, self-esteem	14 (11.1)
Support from family/friends	10 (7.9)
Compliance with medication/treatment programmes	6 (4.8)
Suitable employment	4 (3.2)
Total responses	126 (100.0)

asked staff for their perception of the factors that impeded or promoted the residents' return to independent living.

9.2.1 Profile of respondents

A total of 52 staff from the sampled residences completed questionnaires. Of these, 65% worked in high support residences, 19% were in medium support residences and 15% were in low support residences. Seventy-one per cent of the staff were female. Table 9.2 presents the professional status of the staff, by level of support. The majority of staff in the high support residences were mental health nurses (85%) as were the majority of the low support staff (87%). The majority of staff allocated to the medium support residences (70%) were care workers or care assistants, while 30% were mental health nurses. While no mental health nursing staff worked within individual medium or low support residences, there were nursing officers in charge of these residences. Their role is to oversee the residences and monitor the health and wellbeing of the residents.

Most of the staff surveyed were on permanent contracts (88%) and in full-time employment (81%). Only 15% of staff were employed on a part-time basis, with two members of staff job sharing. The majority of the staff (58%) were mental health professionals for 16 years or more, with 38% employed as mental health professionals for 26 years or more. Only 10% were employed for five years or less, and 21% were employed for ten years or less at the time of the study. The length of time in the current post was five years or less for 48% of the respondents, while 40% were in their current post between 6 and 16 years. A total of 11% of respondents did not answer the question. These results suggested that the majority of the staff surveyed were highly experienced mental health nurses.

9.2.2 Perceived aims and functions of community residences

Staff of the residences surveyed were asked to rate eight variables (scale of 1 - 3) relating to the importance of the aims and functions of the residence. Table 9.3 shows the eight possible functions and the number and percentage of staff reporting their perception of the importance of each function.

A large number of staff perceived the community residences as having a function in the rehabilitation of residents so that they might progress to lower levels of support or independent living (90%). As Table 9.3 shows, the majority of staff perceived the residences as providing a psychosocial rehabilitation function and as providing support to residents. Over three-quarters (77%) of staff also perceived the residences as being highly important in terms of providing a home for life (Table 9.3). A total of 54% of the staff perceived that the community residence was of high importance in providing a service to shorten inpatient treatment, and 52% perceived it as central to providing an alternative to inpatient care. Fifty per cent of the staff reported that community residences were important in providing respite care. Forty per cent of staff stressed the complementary function of community residences as an adjunct to other elements of services (i.e. outpatient / day care / home care), while 44% of staff perceived the community residences as important for the provision of care during crisis.

9.3 STAFF PERCEPTIONS OF FACTORS THAT PROMOTED INDEPENDENT LIVING

Staff were asked to identify the three most important factors that they felt promoted independent behaviour. The researcher categorised responses into eight main categories. Table 9.4 shows the eight categories and the number of responses in each category. The percentage of the total responses is provided in brackets. The number of responses does not refer to the number of staff, as staff provided more than one response to the questions. Table 9.4 presents the categories in the order of the frequency of responses.

Staff frequently reported 'support from the staff' (21%) as an important factor in the promotion of independent living. Responses that fell into this category concerned well-trained staff who were encouraging, trustworthy, and respectful and provided a good atmosphere or environment for residents. In addition, staff highlighted the importance of choice, privacy and an independent environment for residents:

☐ *supportive / dynamic multi-disciplinary team*

☐ *team that allows for and knows individual differences*

☐ *well trained staff who show interest in client*

☐ *open-minded staff, consistent approach, committed and genuinely care*

☐ *environment that encourages choice, privacy, independent environment*

A total of 21% of the staff responses was categorised into the independence, choice and participation category. The staff perceived participation in decision making, acceptance of responsibility for personal care and having a level of independence and choice as important factors in promoting independent living.

☐ *give residents responsibility*

☐ *taking control of personal activities – medication and household chores*

☐ *taking charge of their own money*

☐ *active participation in decision making regarding their care plans*

☐ *autonomy*

☐ *making decisions for themselves*

A total of 17% of responses from the staff addressed the importance of community support and involvement in the promotion of independent living. Staff felt that residents need more integration into the community in the form of social activities and other community schemes such as worklink.

Table 9.5   Number (%) of responses in each category of factors believed to impede independent living*

Categories

Staff and health care team – lack of training, lack of encouragement, lack of interest, not multi-disciplinary	23
Lack of independence, responsibility, participation, decisions	16
Illness – severe symptoms, relapse, re-admissions, fear of relapse	11
Lack of support from community, family, friends	10
Routine – too much, monotony	6
Apathy, negativity of individual	9
Poor compliance with medication / treatment programmes	8
Institutionalisation	8
Lack of training, education and rehabilitation of patient	6
Inadequate personal finances	6
Total	103

* Note; more than one response was provided by staff to this question

☐ *community acceptance and involvement*

☐ *going to pictures, days out and trying to get back into community as best as possible*

☐ *support with other community disciplines and systems – worklink etc.*

☐ *integration and involvement in the community*

A total of 14% of the responses of staff recognised the importance of training, education, guidance and rehabilitation in promoting independent living. These responses referred mainly to rehabilitation programmes and included:

☐ *education in daily living skills*

☐ *guidance*

☐ *behavioural therapy interventions*

☐ *occupational work or training*

☐ *rehabilitation and relearning*

☐ *individualised training programmes*

☐ *rehabilitation process*

Only 11% (n = 14) of staff responses referred to the importance of confidence and self-esteem in promoting independent living. For example, responses referred to 'confidence building', 'bolster self-esteem' and 'high self-esteem' as important factors in promoting independent living. A total of 8% of responses reported family and friends support as the important factors to promote independent living. Compliance with medication was mentioned in only 5% (n = 6) of staff responses, while suitable employment was mentioned in only 3% (n = 4) of responses.

9.4   FACTORS PERCEIVED TO HAVE IMPEDED INDEPENDENT LIVING

Staff responses to the factors that impeded independent living best fitted within ten categories. Table 9.5 shows these response categories and the number of responses in each category. Categories are ordered by frequency of responses. There were 103 responses regarding factors that impede return to independent living.

The most frequently reported response had to do with staff and health care team. A total of 22% of responses were relevant to this category. Responses referred to the lack of staff training, lack of encouragement, lack of interest and non-multidisciplinary work practices as factors impeding independence.

"staff doing too much for clients"

"staff not interested"

"lack of training for staff, specifically for rehab purposes"

"lack of understanding and patience"

"lack of multidisciplinary intervention"

The second most frequent factor perceived by staff as impeding return to integrated living in the community was lack of independence of the resident. This included lack of responsibility, lack of participation in treatment and care and non-involvement in decision making. Some examples of the responses in this category included:

"rigid thinking, restrictive, judgemental approaches from staff"

"too much medication"

"no individual or personal responsibility"

"no participation in decision making process regarding their care plans"

"not letting people do things for themselves"

A total of 11% of the responses referred to the illness and the severity of the illness as factors that impeded return to independent living. These responses referred specifically to severe and recurring symptoms. For example, recurring symptoms, addiction and drug abuse were specially mentioned."

A total of 10% of the responses reported that the lack of support from the community, families and friends hindered the residents' return to independent living.

Nine per cent of the responses referred to apathy and lack of motivation of the resident as impeding return to independent living. Other factors that were mentioned less frequently included institutionalisation (8%), and poor compliance with medication and treatment programmes (8%), routine and monotony (6%), lack of training and rehabilitation (6%) and inadequate personal finances (6%).

9.5 SUMMARY

Of staff who responded to the questionnaires, the majority were female and mental health nurses. They had been employed as mental health professionals for some time and most had permanent contracts.

Regarding the aims and functions of the residences, the staff perceived that the residences had an important role to play in the rehabilitation of the residents to independent living or towards lower levels of support. However, a large proportion of the staff felt that the residences also had an important role in providing a 'home for life' for the residents. The results suggested that staff viewed the residences as having a dual purpose – rehabilitation and long term care. It was also interesting to note that half of the staff perceived the residences as having a function in the care and treatment of the patients to complement other mental health service components such as inpatient, respite and crisis care. It was clear that the staff did not view the residences as filling just one function, but rather as filling a number of important and diverse functions.

Factors most frequently perceived as promoting independent living were support from the staff, independence and autonomy of the residents and community support and involvement. It is clear that the staff felt that they had an important role in helping and supporting the residents achieve independent living. This they perceived was helped by giving the resident independence, choice, responsibility and encouragement to participate in all areas of their lives. Likewise the most frequently reported factor considered by staff as impeding return to independent living was lack of staff training in rehabilitation, lack of encouragement, lack of interest and non-multidisciplinary teams. In addition, dependency of the resident, be it either through their own choice or through the over provision of care and support from the staff, was perceived as an impediment to returning to integrated living in the community. Severity of illness and relapse were also frequently considered by staff as factors that impeded return to independent living while inadequate personal finance was perceived only by approximately 6% of staff as a factor that prevented the return of the residents to integrated living.

CHAPTER 10
Life in Community
Residences: Conclusion and
Discussion

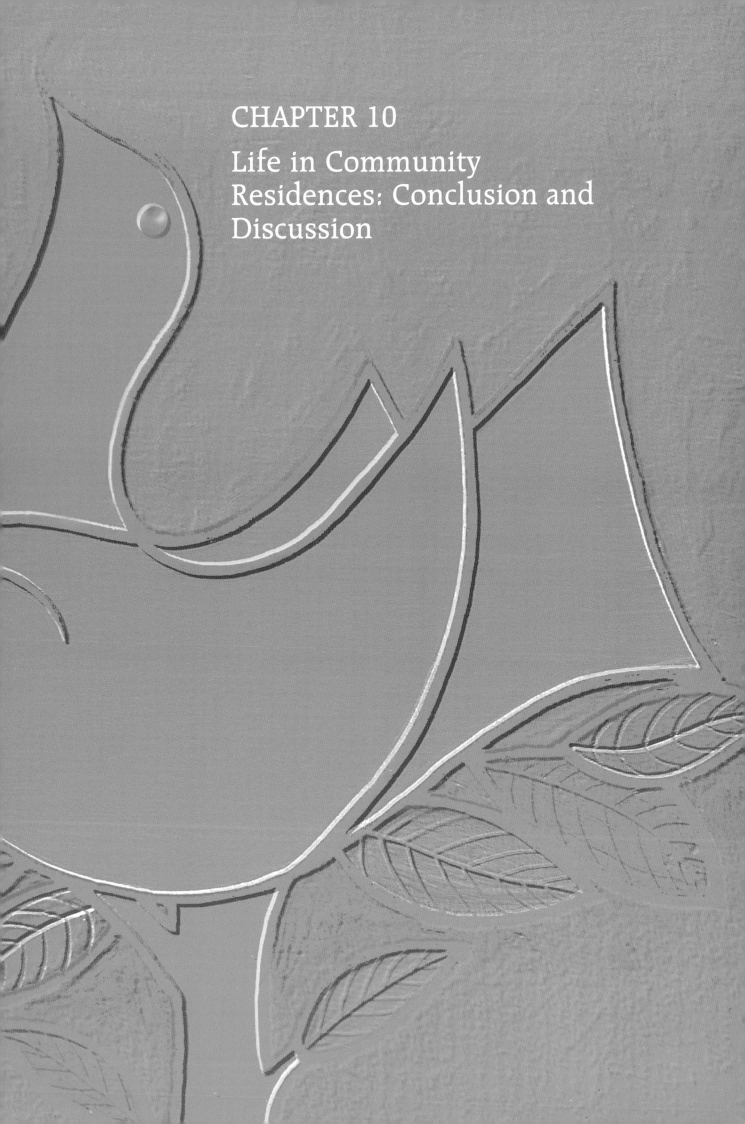

Chapter 10

Life in community residences: conclusion and discussion

The present study was carried out in response to significant changes in mental health policy and the lack of mental health services research in community residential care In Ireland. The study aimed to review the provision, functions and purposes of community residential services. Of primary importance were the residents' views of the treatment and care provided by mental health services and their perceptions of their lives. The study set out to determine where community residential care was provided, what care was provided, to whom it was provided and satisfaction levels of residents and the extent to which the service was meeting residents' needs. Finally, the study sought to determine whether those in community residential care were appropriately placed and, if not, what alternative care would best meet their needs.

To provide an overall picture of community residential care, Chapter 10 will amalgamate the findings presented in the previous chapters and discuss these results in terms of the nature and quality of community residential accommodation and the extent to which it met the needs of the residents. Based on the study findings, a series of recommendations is made in Chapter 11.

10.1 RESIDENCES AND THE RESIDENTS

This study was primarily quantitative in its emphasises, but included a series of open-ended questions which were analysed in order to illustrate residents' and staff views about different aspects of care. Many positive findings have come out of the questionnaires as to how the residents viewed their lives and the perceived independence and control they had in leading their lives as they wished. The findings have shown that, in general, the majority of the residents were satisfied with their current accommodation and treatment and care. The perception of life in the residences was positive and self-reports of quality of life rated it as high. In general, the residents felt that they had control over their lives and were happy with their level of independence. However, residents were also asked open-ended questions regarding their lives and their current accommodation. Their responses qualified and elaborated on their views of their lives. For example, although residents

reported that they were happy in their current accommodation, this may have been a result of their perceptions that they had no where else to go. Given the lack of the provision of more independent accommodation to meet the needs of these residents, such perceptions were accurate. In addition, residents reported that, if things could be changed, they would like more independence in terms of being able to cook and eat when and what they liked and to spend their money as they pleased. While many residents appeared to know what money they received each week, many received help to manage their finances. The researcher noted during site visits that most residents were not concerned about handing control of their finances to nursing staff and did not take responsibility for their own finances, nor, in fact, did they feel they had the skills to do so. However, a number of residents did feel that they should have control of their own money and wanted to spend it as they saw fit. Many of the residents had previous inpatient admissions for long periods of time and, in fact, many had been relocated from the large psychiatric hospitals. Many, therefore, had spent long periods of time in a culture of dependency and guardianship, as opposed to one of independence and control. It is possible that residents failed to see the possibility for change in a system that they had become accustomed to for the best part of their lives. In addition, as the majority of staff had been in the system for long periods of time, they also may have failed to see the system as one that emphasised recovery as opposed to maintenance. These results highlight the need for training and education for all in community residential facilities in the competencies and principles of recovery. These points will be reiterated and qualified throughout the discussion as appropriate.

Before addressing the occupancy of the residences and the care and treatment provided it is necessary to highlight the characteristics of the residents in terms of their socio-demographic and clinical profile and the level of support that was provided.

10.1.1 Level of support provided in community residences

Residential accommodation for people with mental health problems in Ireland is provided on three levels of support – high, medium and low support. An important point to note is that these levels of support were not uniformly defined throughout the study areas, nor are they, in fact, on a national level. High support residences throughout the country are standardised in that all provide 24-hour nursing. However, definitions of medium support and low support vary. Medium support in some areas included night-time supervision, while in others no supervision at night was provided. Low support was generally standardised, with regular visits from staff. However, in some areas staff visited on a daily basis while in others staff visited on a weekly basis. Concern regarding the variation in the definition of levels of support in a national context was expressed on a number of occasions by the management and staff of the residences. For the purposes of this research the following definitions were used as these are the most common definitions of the three levels of support:

□ High support – 24-hour nursed care

□ Medium support – night-time supervision by non-nursing staff

□ Low support – regular visits by staff

These definitions equate with those in the UK (Lelliott et al., 1996; Donnelly et al., 1994) in that high support have 24-hour nursed care and low support are not staffed, but have regular staff visits. However, in the U.K., medium support facilities are staffed 24-hours, with staff sleeping at night-time.

10.1.2 A profile of the sample of residents

The average age of the residents in community residences was 53 years, with the majority between the ages of 46 and 65 years. Few were under the age of 35 years and almost one-third were over the age of 65 years. A slightly higher proportion of the residents were male and both genders were equally represented in the interviews. Most of the residents were single and approximately half had attended secondary school, with only a quarter having post-secondary or third-level education.

Similarly to previous research in residential care (Lelliott et al., 1996; de Girolamo et al., 2002; Donnelly et al., 1996) the majority of the residents had a diagnosis of schizophrenia and had a long duration of illness. The majority of residents had previous inpatient hospitalisations; however, there were few admissions reported over the previous five years. This corresponded to the clinical symptoms reported for residents who were interviewed, with the majority experiencing mild symptoms. In addition, few residents showed moderate or severe impairments in clinical functioning in the previous two weeks. It would appear that symptoms had been relatively stable for some time. The course of illness for the majority of residents in the previous five years was persistent, but stable, and there were no significant differences between those in high, medium and low support residences.

In terms of the general level of occupational and social functioning (GAF), the high support residents generally had lower levels of functioning; however, the clinical significance of these differences is questionable. The mean scores of all groups were above 40 (scores less than 40 indicate a marked degree of disability (de Girolamo et al., 2004).

Difficulties were reported as moderate for the high support residents, while mild difficulties were reported for the medium and low support residents. On average, few problems with clinical and social functioning were reported for the residents in the two weeks prior to interview, while, slightly more were reported as having experienced mild to moderate problems in activities of daily living and occupation (HoNOS). This is in line with previous research that indicated that those in residential accommodation had relatively high skills level (Donnelly et al., 1996). Interestingly, Donnelly et al., (1996) found that highly staffed accommodation could result in a deterioration of skills, specifically self-care skills. This suggests that over-providing for the residents may actually be detrimental to their move towards independence. This notion has also being highlighted by residents themselves in that they viewed lack of encouragement from staff to do things for themselves as an important factor that impeded the return to independence. An interesting finding was that residents rated themselves as functioning at a higher level than that rated by key workers, although there was a significant positive correlation, albeit weak, between the two ratings. Two possible explanations are presented as to why this would occur. This finding could be due to the over-estimation by the residents of their own functioning or the under-estimation of the key workers of the residents' functioning. It has been shown that stigma surrounding mental illness may also be present in mental health care professionals (Hocking, 2003). The key workers ratings may be influenced by their low expectations of the residents arising from the lack of training in recovery and rehabilitation and previous experience of working in a system that aspired to maintenance of current skills and abilities as

opposed to development and recovery. This issue requires further research.

In contrast to the study by Lelliott et al., (1996) in the UK, the majority of residents in high, medium and low support were not experiencing physical health problems. In fact, few residents had severe physical health disabilities with only a very small proportion having mild to moderate problems most commonly in the metabolic / endocrine system and cardiovascular and digestive disabilities. This most likely reflects the younger age profile of the residents interviewed in this study, which is more comparable with that of residents in the Italian study (de Girolamo et al., 2002) than those in the UK study (Lelliott et al., 1996).

In summary, the residents in this sample showed a low rate of clinical symptoms and generally had good physical health. In addition, their general occupational and social functioning was above the level that indicates marked disability. This brings into question the need for the levels of care and support provided to these residents and would argue that the needs of the residents are over-provided for in terms of the clinical and physical needs. However, as will be discussed further on, other needs are clearly not being met, such as independent living and rehabilitation, suggesting that the current levels of service provision are not appropriately targeted to meet the specific needs of some residents. This undermines the principle of recovery whereby individuals are empowered to take control of their lives.

10.2 COMMUNITY RESIDENTIAL PLACES AND OCCUPANCY RATE

There were 102 residences reported for the three HSE local areas, providing a total of 951 residential places. This represented a rate of 96 places per 100,000 total population in the areas studied.

10.2.1 Rate of places

The majority of these places were in 24-hour-staffed residences (584) with a smaller number in medium support (166) and low support (201) residences. The *Report of the Inspector of Mental Health Services* (MHC, 2005a) pointed out that variation existed within Ireland in the rate of 24-hour-staffed residential places per 100,000 population with the highest at approximately 190 per 100,000 and the lowest at 8 places per 100,000. The average rate of places in high support residences in the three areas studied was 76 per 100,000 adult population, ranging from 85 places per 100,000 in Area B, 77 places per 100,000 in Area A and 36 places per 100,000 in Area C. The development of residential facilities was based on the existence of psychiatric hospitals and deinstitutionalisation, as opposed to a population needs-based approach. It had been highlighted by the Inspector of Mental Hospitals (Department of Health and Children, 2004) that areas where large psychiatric hospitals existed had the highest number of 24-hour-staffed residential places. There were large psychiatric hospitals located in all areas studied, three of which had been closed completely, one had 20 patients remaining and three hospitals catered for approximately 318 patients in total. The area that had the lowest rate of residential places was indeed the area where the psychiatric hospitals had not yet been closed (i.e. Area C) and catered for the greatest number of patients. While high rates of places may have been necessary during the programme of deinstitutionalisation, the continued need for so many high support places is questionable. As the number of individuals relocated from psychiatric hospitals decreased so too should the number of high support places. There is a concern that the availability of places may lead to the admission of those who could be better provided for in their own environment. A needs-based approach to planning is necessary. This will ensure that the best care is provided to service users in their own environment and that a sufficient number of high support places is available for those in need of high levels of care.

The planning norm recommended for 24-hour-staffed residences in *A Vision for Change* was 30 places per 100,000 in large urban areas and fewer places in areas with low deprivation levels. It must be noted that this figure was an estimate for the number of high support residential places required for the future. In two of the participating areas, the number of high support residences far exceeded this estimate (77 places per 100,000 and 85 places per 100,000), while the area that had not completely closed the large psychiatric hospitals had a rate of places similar to that recommended in *A Vision for Change* (36 places per 100,000). In addition, *A Vision for Change* recommends that 120 intensive-care rehabilitation places should be provided nationally and 80 places in high support intensive-care residences. In addition, *A Vision for Change* recommended that 130 places nationally should be provided as crisis places. Thus, with the inclusion of these residential places, two of the areas in the current study have close to the recommended provision of places necessary for various forms of high support, while one area requires the provision of more high support places. It is necessary to note that, while the number of places in high support is close to the recommended number, the aims and functions of these residences may change.

10.2.1.1 High support

On a national level a census in 2006 indicated that there were 1,412 persons resident in high support residences (Tedstone Doherty *et al.*, in press). The number of places in high support residences was 1,383 in 2003 (Department of Health and Children, 2004). If we take, as recommended in *A Vision for Change*, 30 high support places per 100,000 population with 10 places in each unit, this results in a total of 1170 places nationally. When a further 120 intensive-care rehabilitation places, the 80 places in high support intensive-care residences and the 130 places in crisis residences are added this comes to 1500 community-based high support places, which is similar to that now provided, even if the latter three categories are not strictly comparable in purpose with the bulk of non-specialised high support community-based accommodation. The inevitable conclusion is that, if demand quantitatively remains as it is, there will be little change in high support accommodation either in physical provision or in staffing levels, and, therefore, little saving for the mental health services through reduced high support provision. Indeed, the reduction in size of the high support residences to ten places, as advocated in *A Vision for Change*, may require an increase in staffing numerically. Whereas the clientele of the present high support residences was largely drawn from the psychiatric hospital old long-stay population, whose characteristics are well known, this accommodation in the future will be required for younger, new long-stay people. These people will not be long-stay in the hospital sense, but long-stay in the sense of having newly derived persistent illness, mainly psychotic, with housing needs. There is an uncertainty about the characteristics and needs of this newly accruing population, many of whom are likely to have co-morbid

substance abuse and may be less likely to settle easily into high support accommodation than their elder peers who were institutionalised for many years before being moved to community settings. This newer group is already beginning to increase in numbers and information on their needs has to be retrospectively and prospectively accumulated to guide further high support planning. So, while there may be enough residences in terms of quantity, the aims and functions and the quality of these residences need to be addressed.

It must also be borne in mind that it has been recommended that the public psychiatric hospitals close as soon as possible (*A Vision for Change*; MHC 2006c). These hospitals cater for approximately 774 long-stay patients, of whom over half are 65 years or over. With the closure of these hospitals, alternative community-based residential accommodation of varying levels of support for the more active and mobile of these patients, who constitute the majority, will be required. For those whose physical health is compromised or who have severe mobility or cognitive problems, nursing home placement will be necessary. A similar consideration also applies to current residents in community residences with similar disabilities.

10.2.1.2 Medium and low support

It is the medium and, particularly, the low support places, of which there were approximately 1,827 in 2003 (Department of Health and Children, 2003) that pose particular concern. It would seem from the recommendations of *A Vision for Change* that local authorities should provide housing for this group, but the practicalities and the reality of implementing this recommendation needs to be addressed. For example, and not especially encouraging indications of why this may fail to be realised, are the facts already set out in Chapter 2 – the extent of the waiting lists, the fact that the residents are considered by housing authorities to be housed, that they do not in general constitute family units, that some are quite elderly and that, even if the authorities did provide housing, are suspect that the mental health services would not provide the necessary care. Furthermore it is the low and medium support residents who show the greatest potential for independent living.

One possible solution is to induce local housing authorities to take possession of low support residences in so far as their administration and maintenance requirements are concerned. This would fulfil their commitment as set out in the 2005 Housing Policy Framework – Building Sustainable Communities – to the extent that special needs would be met for those with disabilities including psychiatric disabilities. There should be a commitment that this housing stock remains exclusively for the use of persons with mental health problems. This entails a partnership approach with the mental health services providing the necessary level of care. As far as ensuring that residents become tenants of the local authority in the true sense of that word, the provisions of the 2004 Residential Tenancy Act need to be fulfilled (i.e. security of tenure, periods of notice, registration). Side by side with this are the innovative tenancy training schemes and the newly derived initiative by local authorities in setting up new tenancy arrangements with landlords in a mutually sustainable partnership such as is being promoted by the Tenancy Sustainable Group.

As far as medium support accommodation is concerned, greater involvement of voluntary agencies, such as has already been achieved by Respond, HAIL, STEER and local mental health associations, should be encouraged, with greater involvement in the procurement of properties and in the organisation, management and maintenance of such settings jointly with residents themselves, and a retraction of the psychiatric professional presence other than in a care and clinical support and rehabilitative capacity. It should be borne in mind that many local mental health associations are heavily representative of mental health professionals.

The provision of housing and care is further addressed in Section 10.3, giving examples of alternative models of provision in the UK and in Ireland.

10.2.2 Occupancy rate

At the time of the study there were 871 residents in the residences. Based on the number of residents in places, the occupancy rate was 92%. However, this did not reflect the 76 places designated for other uses (i.e. respite and crisis care). Thus, inclusion of these places resulted in an occupancy rate of almost full capacity (i.e. 99.6%). While only 8% of the places were reported by nursing officers as designated respite or crisis places, interviews with staff confirmed that a significant number perceived that the provision of respite care was an important function of the community residential facilities. As highlighted in *A Vision for Change*, the use of community residential places for other purposes such as respite or crisis care must be questioned especially in terms of the sensitivities of the core residents of the facility. The use of places for these purposes may impact negatively on the care and treatment of the residents by disturbing their social environment or by distracting staff from their primary function of providing therapeutic activities for the core residents. *A Vision for Change* recommended that additional places be provided for crisis care, recommending 130 places nationally.

10.3 PROVISION OF RESIDENTIAL ACCOMMODATION AND CARE

The majority of the high support residences were large renovated houses in private grounds and were owned by the HSE. The majority of the medium and low support residences were also owned by the HSE and were semi-detached houses situated in housing estates. Sixteen of the low support residences were leased from private owners. These findings confirmed that mental health services are the primary providers of accommodation for those with persistent mental health problems and housing needs.

10.3.1 Lack of alternative accommodation

As highlighted in Section 2.6.5.1, there was no policy in place that specifically addressed housing needs for those with mental health problems. Residents were entitled to go on the local authority waiting lists and it was reported by nursing officers that many were on these lists and had been for some time. As mentioned above, social housing continues to be based on a points system, resulting in those with children being giving priority for housing. The high number of single persons in community residences, coupled with the under-provision of social housing at a national level, has in the past resulted in few housing alternatives for people in community residences in mental health services.

In line with previous findings, the desire for alternative independent living was reflected in the comments made by the residents (Shepherd, 1998). While the majority of residents were happy in their current accommodation, some commented that if given the choice they would like to have their own home. A number said that they would like their own accommodation, but had nowhere else to go. Residents reported that they had been on the local authority housing waiting list for some years (one resident reported a seven year waiting period) and felt that they had no hope of getting local authority accommodation in the near future. In addition, while residents reported that they would like their own home, many also expressed a need for support. In a review of the literature, Shepherd (1998) found that the majority of people would prefer their own homes, even though they acknowledged the need for flexible support. The residents in this study felt that independent accommodation would result in the loss of needed support and, consequently, they were best placed in their current accommodation. A significant number of residents had no alternative option that met their current housing need and also provided the necessary supports, both medical and psycho-social. Management in community residences reported that they felt the responsibility for housing should be the sole responsibility of the local housing authorities and not mental health services.

10.3.2 Non-statutory agencies and the provision of housing

Given the current shortage of social housing in Ireland, what alternative models of provision are available? Alternative models for housing provision for those with mental health difficulties have been outlined in Section 2.6.5.2. One such model implemented in the UK, termed Registered Social Landlords, provides residential facilities. Previously, these social landlords provided housing with external agencies such as voluntary agencies providing management and care practices.

More recently, there has been a move towards social landlords providing both management and care services. However, a number of problems with this model have been identified. Firstly, training of staff responsible for management and care has been criticised, with the majority of staff poorly trained and the self-reporting of unmet training needs (Senn *et al*, 1997). Secondly, there has been a bias towards the selection of clients thought to be more 'easily' treated (Shepherd & Murray, 2001). And thirdly, the monitoring of these facilities in terms of quality of care and best practice has been criticised (Shepherd & Murray, 2001). A code of standards in the provision of housing and support for people with mental health problems, and a guide on how to achieve these standards, have been produced in the UK (NHF/MHF, 1996; Warner *et al.*, 1997). The first step towards realising this model of provision in Ireland would be the establishment of effective partnerships and close interagency co-operation, so that a planned and informed approach could be developed from the outset, ensuring quality and good practice.

10.3.3 Local housing associations and voluntary groups

Within Ireland, a small number of local housing associations have been formed by voluntary agencies such as STEER and HAIL with grant aid from the Department of the Environment, Heritage and Local Government. An example of a recent project which aims to address the provision of affordable social housing for people with mental health problems is the STEER Housing Association. This is currently being developed in one of the study areas and aims to provide secured tenancies with appropriate levels of support for client groups. The project will provide one, two and three bedroom dwellings to meet the housing needs of a diverse range of potential clients in both urban and rural settings. 'Recovery guides' will be available to provide tenants with non-medical interventions to maintain and promote positive mental health and for the maintenance of the tenancy. The trained 'recovery guides' will be past or present service users and will provide low to medium levels of support. Each housing scheme will have a communal centre that will be staffed both morning and night to provide the required level of support to tenants as and when it is needed. The centre will be used for social events and for the provision of courses and training on social and life skills. This model of housing and care provision is based on the recovery model of care (Anthony, 1993) emphasising independence, dignity and support, following consultation with service users. The model values the concept of the individual having their own home and at the same time the necessary supports to ensure self-confidence and self-efficacy. This model of provision will be piloted in one of the HSE areas of the study. It is envisaged that this housing will not entirely replace the current model of housing and care provision (i.e. HSE provision of high, medium and low support), but rather will be a part of a range of options that clients can avail of to suit their needs. It is imperative that this model of housing and care provision is evaluated from the outset taking into consideration the health service management, service users and care providers perspectives. This will ensure that quality and best practice prevail and also the identification of those best suited to this type of care. This model should be assessed as a possible model of housing and care provision to be provided on a national basis. Other models of housing provision by local housing associations and voluntary groups around the country should also be evaluated as above.

10.3.4 The way forward

It is clear from the findings of the current study that the provision of housing for those with persistent mental health problems has long been the responsibility of the mental health services. This has been the result of the lack of social housing provision by local authorities, especially during deinstitutionalisation programmes. Many of the residents interviewed had no alternative but to avail of community residential care. Yet many voiced their desire and hope to live in a less clinical community setting, based in ordinary housing. There is a need within Ireland to provide a more comprehensive range of residential facilities for those with severe and persistent mental illness than that currently provided. Such facilities are needed to provide for different levels of functioning. It is envisaged that they will include housing with high levels of clinical support (e.g. 24-hour nursed care) and more independent settings with supports available when needed and preferably provided by non-clinically trained 'recovery guides'. As suggested in *A Vision for Change*, only a small number of high support places will be necessary in each local area. The majority of people should be supported in ordinary housing. The provision of housing should not be the responsibility of the mental health services and, thus, there is an urgent need for mental health services to collaborate with local housing authorities and voluntary bodies to identify needs and requirements in local areas. For these partnerships to work effectively, there needs to be mutual understanding and respect between the agencies in relation to their respective roles and responsibilities.

10.4 THE ENVIRONMENTAL FEATURES AND CLIMATE AND CULTURE OF THE RESIDENCES

The internal environment, management style and climate and culture of the community residential facilities can impact on the residents' satisfaction (Rog, 2004). Of particular importance is respect for the individual and the principle of informed choice (Schizophrenia Ireland, 2006). A 'client orientated' management style, involving high levels of positive staff-client interactions, is likely to contribute to the residents' wellbeing. An authoritarian regime which denies basic rights and privacy is not conducive to the residents' wellbeing particularly when they are subjected to unnecessary rules and regulations (Shephard & Murray, 2001). Quality of care indices in residential facilities have included quality of the physical environment, individualisation of care, privacy, autonomy and the attractiveness of the neighbourhood (Shepherd, 2000; Schizophrenia Ireland, 2006). Few residences in the current study had evaluation and review plans for monitoring the quality of services provided.

10.4.1 The aims and functions of the residences

It was reported by management and clinical staff that, initially, the community residences were viewed as 'homes for life' by both staff and residents. However they felt that as the deinstitutionalisation programme advanced and within the current climate of change in the mental health services, the aims and functions of the residences were changing to one of rehabilitation and recovery. There was concern voiced as to the situation of those who have lived in community residences for long periods of time. It was felt that moving them, possibly away from familiar friends and neighbourhoods, would cause unnecessary distress to this ageing population. The concept of a 'home for life' was also seen as an important aim of the residences by the staff working in them. These findings reflected the dual role of the residences as one of long term care for some and as a rehabilitation and as a stepping stone to more independent living for others. This was evident also in the comments by residents, with some hoping to complete the remainder of their lives in the residences while others had hopes of moving to more independent living and getting a place of their own. This begs the question – can these facilities perform this dual role effectively to meet the needs of those concerned? Does the prolonged care of some residents hinder the intensive rehabilitation required by others to move to lower levels of support? It is possible that having such a diverse group of people with different needs in the same residence does not help to tailor the treatment and care provided to individuals. In addition, the role of the nursing and care staff is divided between providing continuing care to some and intensive rehabilitation to others. The lack of a co-ordinating rehabilitation team further increases the difficulty, a point made in the recent report of the Inspector of Mental Health Services (MHC, 2006c). There is a need to redefine the aims and functions of community residential facilities. While there is a need for a national definition of the type of care provided, within this definition, local need should determine the use of the current residential facilities.

10.4.2 *Internal environment*

The current study assessed the internal environment of the residences in terms of the staffing levels, sleeping arrangements and number of bathrooms. On average, there were 15 residents in high support residences, six in medium support residences and four in low support residences. Within the high support residences there was on average a ratio of staff to residents

of one to seven for daytime and one to nine at nighttime. In line with previous research, this nursing level would seem particularly high, especially as residents psycho-social functioning and psychopathology was not problematic (Donnelly et al., 1997). The employment of highly skilled nursing staff for administrative or basic tasks may not be the best way in which to deploy valuable resources. While it may be necessary to have two staff present in the residences at any time in case of emergency, one nursing staff member and one care staff member may be sufficient. In addition, with an average of 15 residents in high support residences, it is more likely to resemble a large institution as opposed to a small residence that creates a more home-like environment (MHC, 2006c). *A Vision for Change* recommended that residences should cater for a maximum of 10 residents. Picardi et al., (2005) argued that the size and staffing pattern and skill mix can influence the residents' quality of life. For example, similar to this Picardi *et al.,* (2005) found that many of the residential facilities in Italy did not have access to those professionals that would be expected to have more skill in providing psychosocial rehabilitation. Many of the nursing staff in the residences in this study were providing these rehabilitative interventions without the proper training. This can cause stress both for the nursing staff and residents, which can impact negatively on mental health.

The size of the residence appeared to be related to the possibility of having a single room. The smaller, medium and low support residences had a greater number of single rooms than the high support residences. In most cases, residents shared twin rooms. Whenever possible, residents were able to choose who they shared with, but this was often not possible. This inability to provide residents with a single room impacted on their privacy and was reflected in comments by the residents. One resident made reference to the fact, that while the community residence was better than the streets, there was no privacy. However some residents also commented that they liked having a room-mate. This highlighted the different needs of residents and the importance of choice. The importance of choice in mental health services was also made in a recent report of service –users' views (Schizophrenia Ireland, 2006). The lack of bathrooms and showers was also highlighted in the current study. The high ratio of residents to bathrooms is unacceptable and en-suite bathrooms should be available, as is now the norm in many homes. The privacy of en-suite bathrooms is even more imperative for people who are unrelated and who share accommodation. The planning of smaller residences with single rooms and en-suites will improve the privacy and comfort of the residents.

In this study 29% of the residences did not provide residents with access to public phones making communication with family and friends difficult. It was reported that residents could use the office phone; however, this again was detrimental to the privacy of the resident and increased their dependency on staff. The ownership of mobile phones was not addressed in the study and a number of residents may have owned a mobile phone.

Service managers, clinical directors and directors of nursing pointed out that residential accommodation was mainly purchased on an ad-hoc basis during the deinstitutionalisation programme and renovated as necessary. During site visits the researcher came across only one specially designed high support residence. This explained the less than ideal situation of many

of the residences. Many of the residences were not suitable for those with mobility problems. This was especially problematic for the ageing population, with nearly a third of all residents being over the age of 65 years. This was highlighted on many of the site visits. Many of the bedrooms in the residences were upstairs and many of the residences, especially the older ones, could not be fitted with lifts. During site visits, the researcher was informed in one instance that the visiting room in one of the residences was currently being used as a bedroom for a resident who was quite ill.

Very few of the residences had evaluation and review plans that monitored the quality of services or the satisfaction of the service users or their families. *A Vision for Change* highlights the importance of service evaluation, especially in terms of quality of life measures and the impact of services on service users and their families. One method for evaluating quality has been the FACE (Functional Assessment of Care Environments) tool which has been used in Northern Ireland as a formal quality evaluation procedure in mental health services (Mc Gilloway *et al.*, 1999).

10.4.3 External environment – accessibility

On average, the residences were located within walking distance of shops, post office and GP surgery, with the distance to the day centre or day hospital somewhat greater. Enquiries about the possession of private transport showed that very few residents owned a car, bike or motorbike. This finding was similar to that found in the Italian study (Santone at al., 2005). The possession of some form of transport is the norm for the majority of people and for the residents it would greatly increase their autonomy and their ability to meet some of their daily needs independently. This may not be especially problematic for those living in urban areas, but for those in rural areas with underdeveloped public transport services, access to transport is a necessity for autonomy and independence. The majority of the high support residences had access to a minibus for transportation, which was mainly used for transporting residents to day centres. Given that the majority of residents did not have access to their own transport, accommodation should be provided in urban areas, close to all amenities.

10.4.4 Climate and culture of the residences: a home-like environment

The philosophy behind the policy was that residential facilities would provide a more home-like environment for residents than that provided in large institutions. This study found that the residences, even the medium and low support residences, were quite restrictive in what the residents were allowed and did not differ significantly in this regard to the large institutions. The institutional design and practice of the 24-hour nursed facilities was also raised in the Report of the Inspector of Mental Health Services (MHC, 2006c). For example, the comings and goings of the residents were often monitored; residents did not have their own door key and could not lock their bedroom doors. In addition, residents did not have access to the kitchen in high support facilities. Even residents in medium and low support facilities often had their food cooked elsewhere (e.g. day centre). While some residents said that they were happy with this situation and made positive comments about the food, others felt that they should have been able to make their own food and have a choice in what they ate. This was exemplified in a comment by one of the residents that it was not good that you couldn't make your own tea and choose what to eat. Health and safety legislation, such as HACCP (see Section 3.3.6), prevents residents from having access to kitchens and it is important that this is revisited in relation to community residences, whereby independence is encouraged and supported. As expected the high support residences were most restrictive in terms of rules and regulations and some of these are in the best interest of the residents for safety reasons. Nevertheless overprotection of residents with unnecessary rules and regulations is not in their best interest and encourages dependency rather than decreasing it, a point previously made by the Department of Health and Children (2003). In times of illness the need to restrict residents' activities for short periods of time may be warranted and should be discussed with the resident. However, the imposition of rules and regulations on all residents regardless of functioning or needs is not beneficial. Donnelly et al., (1996) pointed out that, even if a degree of risk is involved, staff should find ways to encourage residents to partake in activities outside the residences that lead to personal development. The provision of smaller residences would allow for more individualised plans so that the resident and key worker could work together to determine what is in the resident's best interest.

There was close interaction between residents and staff in the residences. Most of the residents were long-term users of mental health services and consequently were well known to staff, with close personal relationships developing over the years. The residents made many positive comments about the nursing staff, with very few making negative comments. The negative comments referred mainly to the 'protective' nature of the nurses' attitudes (i.e. not letting residents do what they want). This lack of choice and the ability to determine one's own treatment was highlighted in a report of the service users' views of mental health services (Schizophrenia Ireland, 2006). The majority of the nurses working in the residences were experienced mental health nurses who had previously been employed in the large psychiatric institutions and their psychiatric training would have been mainly in custodial care. The comments from staff themselves highlighted the importance of staff training and the impact it can have on the return of the resident to independent living. These findings suggest that there is a need to provide staff, both nursing and non-nursing staff, with the necessary training in recovery and rehabilitation. This should include not only the necessary competencies in recovery, but also the underlying principles of recovery that imparts residents the right to control their lives. *A Vision for Change* recommends that all staff working in rehabilitation should be trained in the competencies and principles of recovery.

10.4.5 The main issues

A number of important points arising from the environment and the climate and culture of the residences need reiteration and will need to be addressed in the future. Firstly, the residences were performing a dual function of continuing care on one hand and rehabilitation on the other. Secondly, residences that are not situated close to an efficient public transport service need to be located close to local amenities and services. And finally, the unnecessary rules and regulations of the residences encouraged dependency, as opposed to independence, and these need to be revised.

10.5 REHABILITATION AND RECOVERY

Those with severe and persistent mental illness require a range of rehabilitative measures to address problems that arise as a direct and indirect result of their illness. These have been outlined in Section 2.3. As stated in previous reports (*A Vision for Change*, 2006; Mental Health Commission, 2005b), the principle of recovery should underpin rehabilitation.

10.5.1 Participation in care and treatment

The extent to which the care of an individual is tailored to his or her needs is usually achieved through the use of care plans. These care plans should be constructed, not on behalf of the individual, but rather by the individual and their key worker and, if appropriate, a relative (Schizophrenia Ireland, 2003). The care plan should contain information from a detailed assessment that includes clinical, physical and social functioning, user and carer aspirations, psychiatric risk assessment and management (Royal College of Psychiatrists, 2003). Individual care plans should be regularly reviewed and amended to address the changing needs of the service user. The present study found that the majority of nursing officers reported that care plans were used by the residences and that a key worker system was in place. It was reported by the majority that these care plans contained information on medical treatment and rehabilitation activities of the residents. This was in contrast to the findings from those residents who were interviewed, with the majority reporting that they did not know what a care plan was, were not involved in drawing up the care plan and did not know or were not sure when the care plan would be reviewed. This is an especially worrying finding that needs further investigation as to whether care plans are in fact in place and why the residents cannot identify what the care plan is and when it will be reviewed. This finding suggests that care plans, when in place, involved very little participation by the individuals themselves and suggested that individuals did not have responsibility for their own treatment and recovery. Staff identified the lack of responsibility and participation by the resident in decision-making as an impediment to independent living. Previous research has highlighted the lack of choice in mental health treatment in Ireland and furthermore, the lack of support from mental health professionals when service users' made decisions about their treatment (Schizophrenia Ireland, 2006). This highlighted the lack of a recovery-oriented service. Given the recent policy document that emphasises a move to a recovery-oriented service (*A Vision for Change*) it is critical that all residents have a formal multidisciplinary assessment, are involved in devising their care plan and have access to a designated key worker. It is important that residents are given the responsibility and ownership of their care plan and moreover, provided with the appropriate support to participate in decision-making regarding their treatment.

In the present study, over half of the residents reported that they knew what their medication was for, and just under half reported that they were aware of the possible side effects. Likewise, just over half of the residents felt that the psychiatrist explained their problems to them and kept them informed of their progress. The comments made by the residents suggested that many felt that the psychiatrist did not listen to their concerns or problems, and that the psychiatrist was always right. A number of residents reported that they did not see the psychiatrist often enough and that there was a frequent change of psychiatrist, which they did not feel gave them continuity of care. Over a quarter of the residents reported that they would have liked more information on their problems. In order for residents to make informed choices and participate fully in their care and treatment, they need to have information on all treatment and care options available to them. This information should be provided in an easily understood format explaining pros and cons. Given that the majority of residents had been in mental health services for an extended period of time, one would have expected that they should already have had this information.

10.5.2 Giving residents back control of their lives

The principle of recovery has been proposed for some time but it is only in recent years that it has gathered momentum in Ireland. This principle has moved away from the previous thinking of 'custodial' care and 'doing things to people' to a more person-centred approach which gives people control over their lives and the basic human rights that many people take for granted (*A Vision for Change*, Roberts & Wolfson, 2004). It is clear from the findings of this study, for example the restrictive nature of the residences and the lack of participation by residents in their care and treatment, that the principle of recovery has been poorly embraced or realised in the community residential facilities. For the principle of recovery to underpin mental health services, the re-training and education of many people will be required. Of particular importance to this report are the residents, staff and management responsible for community residences, staff from other agencies such as housing, social benefits and employment, and last but not least, the general public. The need for staff training and re-education in community residences has been previously addressed. Concerning the change of attitude of the service users the *Values for Action Programme* outlined in *A Vision for Change* showed that attitudes of staff and service users changed following completion of the programme. This programme looked at the extent to which a number of valued life experiences (e.g. choice, relationships, independence) were available in the service users' experience of mental health services. Following completion of the programme, comments from staff showed that they felt that their role was enriched and comments from service users indicated that they felt they had regained their self respect. There is a necessity to educate those who are or will work closely with those with severe and persistent problems on the principles of recovery, for example, those in housing authorities and potential employers.

10.5.3 Are residents moving on?

First and foremost, the results from the present study showed that there was little movement of residents to lower levels of support. Only 179 discharges were reported for the previous year and, of these, 43 were to higher levels of support. This resulted in 136 discharges in the past year to lower levels of accommodation – 14% of the total number of places. In addition, the key workers reported that 85% of residents were currently appropriately placed and predicted that in the following six months most would remain in their current residence. This is somewhat in contrast to the key worker reports of few disabilities in the resident's clinical, social, occupational and physical health functioning. These anomalies may be due to the staff perceptions of the residences as 'homes for life', the institutionalised nature of the residences and lack of training in rehabilitation and recovery. As in previous studies in the UK (Trieman *et al.*, 1998) and

Italy (de Girolamo *et al.*, 2005) the turnover of residents was low and the findings would suggest that a model of continuing care predominated, as opposed to a model emphasising rehabilitation, recovery and progression to lower levels of independence.

10.5.4 Lack of rehabilitation and recovery mental health teams

The majority of the residences were reported as providing rehabilitative interventions that have been shown as important in aiding the individual's optimal level of functioning (WHO, 1996). Before discussing the extent to which these interventions were provided it is necessary to highlight that these interventions were provided in most areas without the assistance of a rehabilitation and recovery mental health team. In only three areas were rehabilitation and recovery mental health teams available to services and these were poorly staffed. *A Vision for Change* outlined the necessary staff and skill mix required for an effective rehabilitation and recovery mental health team. It is of utmost importance that these teams are in post as soon as possible, as recommended by *A Vision for Change*. .

10.5.5 Pharmacological treatment

The majority of residents were on prescribed medication. There is concern that some residents were on both atypical and typical anti-psychotic medication. The medication prescribed to residents should be monitored and evaluated to ensure that the appropriate medication and dosage are prescribed at all times and are in line with best practice guidelines. Some residents made comments regarding the lack of information about their medication and their willingness to change or reduce their medication. However, they felt that their opinions were not valued by the doctors. These negative attitudes towards psychiatrists and the lack of information on medication may lead to less co-operation and compliance with medication. Of utmost importance is that it infringes on the individual's basic right to decide on their own treatment.

10.5.6 Access to rehabilitative activities

The study results found that the majority of residences were providing activities and training for the residents. These included living skills and social skills training and leisure and physical activity. These were provided either in the residences or in the day centres on a group basis. It is important to note that these programmes should be aimed at the individual's needs and requirements (Anthony *et al.*, 1982, Royal College of Psychiatrists, 2003) as opposed to being offered on a group basis. It has been argued that the provision of group programmes results in maintenance programmes, as opposed to programmes that empower the individual to move to the next level of independence (Anthony *et al.*, 1982). It has been suggested that the quality of the activities to aid return to independent living may impact on the quality of life of the resident (de Girolamo *et al.*, 2005). The current study did not address the quality of the activities in community residence. There is a need for further research to address the issue of rehabilitative activities and the impact on the service user's quality of life.

10.5.7 Attendance at day centres / day hospitals

In line with previous research, less than half of the residents were reported as attending a day centre / day hospital (Donnelly *et al.*, 1996). While attendance at a day centre may not be ideal, the low attendance rate brings into question how residents spend their day.

The vast majority of the residents, however, reported that they were not bored during the day. *A Vision for Change* recommends that day centres be available for those who are not in community-based employment or engaged in recreational activities; however, the majority of the interviewed residents were not availing of these options. These findings suggest that many residents were not getting access to rehabilitative activities. The issue of choice must again be reiterated. Many residents may prefer not to attend day centres, and services must provide a range of options, such as the provision of activities in community facilities that include non-users of mental health services. In fact, residents must be actively encouraged to engage in activities that are already provided by community local services and community groups. Furthermore, the quality of the activities in day centres must be evaluated along with the extent to which they meet the needs of the attendees.

10.5.8 Employment options for residents

Only a small number of residences in this study provided vocational training. This is important, as relatively few of the residents interviewed were in paid employment in the community, while a slightly larger number were in sheltered employment. This replicates findings from previous studies in Northern Ireland (Mc Gilloway and Donnelly, 2000). Research has shown that a large proportion of those with severe mental illness want to work in mainstream employment (Bond *et al.*, 2001), a finding that has been replicated in the comments from the residents participating in this study. It was of concern, that only a few of the residences provided activities to encourage work or collaborated with other agencies to find employment. WHO (1996) has argued that training must be provided in a real-world context. The 'place and train' model of employment has been shown to increase the rate of mainstream employment, as opposed to sheltered employment (*A Vision for Change;* Corrigan and McCracken, 2005), and has become the preferred model in the UK and the US (Royal College of Psychiatrists, 2003; Corrigan and McCracken, 2005). These programmes place the individual in mainstream employment and gives them the necessary training and supports relevant to their employment. It must be noted also that meaningful activity is the important factor, be it paid employment, voluntary work or education and skills development (Rankin and Regan, 2004). Mental health services should provide the resident with a range of options so that they can choose those which best suit their needs. A European psychosocial intervention – Assessment Counselling and Coaching in Employment Placement and Training (ACCEPT) aimed at targeting employment was evaluated in Northern Ireland (McGilloway and Donnelly, 2000). This multi-agency programme aimed to provide information, support, training and placement in employment for those whose employability was likely to be affected by mental health problems. The clients of the programme viewed it in a positive light and approximately half were in paid employment or part-time or full-time voluntary work or work experience at the end of the study. Further research is needed to investigate the appropriateness of different models of employment, such as the 'place and train model', within the Irish context.

10.5.9 Psychological support for the residents and their families

WHO (1996) proposes that psychological supports in the form of support and educational services should be provided to service users and their families. This information should include information on rights and the availability of psychosocial resources. In terms of the provision of information to families, less than half of the residences routinely provided family education programmes or had meetings open to relatives. However, it is possible that information was provided to relatives on an informal basis, as a number of staff reported that relatives were welcome to come at any time to discuss issues that concerned them. Staff also suggested that research into the supports needs of the families should be undertaken. While it was not possible address these issues in the current study, the MHRD of the HRB undertook a study to investigate the needs and support requirements of families of relatives with severe and persistent mental illness (Kartalova O'Doherty *et al.,* 2006). In terms of the psychological supports provided to residents, few residences reported that cognitive behavioural therapy was offered. The majority of the residents reported, however, that the key worker was helping them cope with their mental health difficulties and personal problems. In addition, the majority of residents reported that they would seek psychological support from staff during crisis. Regarding the rights of the residents, the majority of the nursing officers reported that residents were given information on their rights, informed about complaints procedures in place and told the name of the local complaints officer. The findings suggest that staff did provide psychological support to residents and that information was provided on rights and complaints procedures, but findings regarding the provision of information to relatives were somewhat less clear.

In terms of support from families and friends, nursing officers reported that a quarter of the residents had no system of support outside of the residences. However, the remainder of the residents had some system of support. Well over half of the residents were reported to have visits from family and friends or went out to visit family and friends. The use of these supports for emotional and practical purposes should be encouraged by staff in the residences. In fact, the residents interviewed reported that they would turn to family and friends as opposed to other residents or staff when needing everyday psychological support.

10.6 ARE RESIDENTS INTEGRATED INTO THE COMMUNITIES IN WHICH THEY LIVE?

Social inclusion refers to the extent to which individuals are part of the community in which they live (Rankin, 2005a). The findings from the current study demonstrated that less than half of the residents attended activities in the community, such as social clubs, bingo, pubs, restaurants and cinemas. The restrictive nature of the residences or the lack of social contacts from outside may have prevented residents from engaging in these activities. Activities to promote community integration, such as activities that involved members of the community, were reported to be provided in the majority of residences; however, this was not reflected in the activities in which residents attended. Previous research has shown that limited social networks can impact negatively on the individual's mental health and use of external services (Becker *et al.*, 1997). It has been suggested that moving activities such as those mentioned earlier (i.e. physical and leisure, training and education) to facilities in communities rather than locating them in day centres, and providing activities that

the wider community can partake can improve community integration for those in residential facilities (Shephard & Murray, 2001). It is important that programmes are individualised and that residents are given choices as opposed to group outings that currently prevail. These large group outings can be stigmatising and are not conducive to integration into the wider community.

10.7 TO WHAT EXTENT DO THE RESIDENTS SHOW INDEPENDENCE?

The residents who participated in the study reported that they were aware of the money they received each week and half said they received help to manage their monies. Yet the nursing officers reported that all residents in medium and low support facilities were capable of managing their own money and only 8% of the high support residents were reported as being unable to manage their own money. This is in sharp contrast to the proportion of those interviewed who were taking control of their finances with no significant differences between those in high, medium or low support residences. The nurses were asked a general question regarding the proportion of residents who could manage their own finances and were not asked about individual residents. A few possible explanations could account for the apparent anomaly in the proportion of residents who were thought able to manage their finances and the actual proportion of residents in the sample who do manage their own money. Firstly, nursing officers may have over-estimated the proportion of the residents that were managing their own finances. Secondly, residents may have been receiving help from others (of which the nurses were unaware), such as family and friends, although this would seem unlikely. And thirdly, while residents may have been able to manage their finances, the institutional culture of the residences may not have encouraged them to do so. The majority of residents went out on their own, yet only two-thirds of high support residents visited the GP by themselves. The majority of residents also reported that they had moderate control over their lives and how they led them and that they were happy with their level of independence. On average, the residents rated their quality of life highly, although those from high support reported a significantly lower quality of life than those from medium or low support residences. The possibility exists that residents do not expect the basic rights that many people take for granted and, given that they have been in the mental health services for a long time, have come to believe that they are incapable of independence. This highlights the importance of expectation and providing residents with competencies and education in the principles of recovery.

10.8 LIMITATIONS OF THE STUDY AND FUTURE RESEARCH

This has been the first comprehensive study in Ireland to evaluate the community residential accommodation for those with severe mental illness. One of the strengths is that it examined life in the residences from the viewpoint of the residents. This is an important aspect of the study and one that provides invaluable information that can be used to design and develop these services in the future.

Given the resources required for such a large scale study on a national level, available resources allowed only three local HSE areas to participate in the current study. The areas were selected based on the number of residences and their willingness to participate. However the authors and advisory group felt that the three areas were generally representative of the community residential mental health services in Ireland in relation to level of development, number of facilities and their location.

While a sufficient number of residents were interviewed for the total sample, the small numbers when stratified by level of support precluded any in-depth sub-group analysis. Furthermore, the sample excluded to a large extent those who moved rapidly through the system, either to independent

living or re-hospitalisation.

Sampling of staff was less than ideal. Given the high turn-over of staff it is difficult to know how representative the sample was. The results suggest that the staff sampled had worked in residential facilities, either inpatient or community, for a long time. Newer staff or those who had worked primarily in community care may have had different perceptions of the community residential facilities. An estimated response rate to the staff questionnaires is provided, however given the fluctuation in staff hours the exact number of staff working in the residence was difficult to estimate.

This study described and evaluated the residential facilities in Ireland. Due to the lack of fully developed rehabilitation teams and services, alternative models of rehabilitation could not be assessed. In addition, the majority of the residential facilities at all levels of support were provided by the mental health services, thus the evaluation of alternative models was not possible. It is important that research and evaluation be carried out on these models as they develop. There is a need to identify which settings are best suited to particular groups of residents and how this improves the quality and appropriateness of care delivered and residents' quality of life.

This study has highlighted a number of areas for further research. Given the low levels of employment of residents, it is not possible to investigate the benefits of various employment models that cater for those in community mental health residential settings within the Irish context. The area of rehabilitation and recovery has received little attention in mental health research. Further research in this area is needed to investigate the process of recovery from the service users' viewpoint. In addition, further research into the psycho-social, cognitive and clinical factors that influence rehabilitation and recovery is required.

10.9 SUMMARY

The aim of this study was to describe the community residential facilities for those with severe mental illness in three HSE local areas in Ireland. While the study investigated only three areas, there is no reason to assume that the range and provision of residential facilities in these areas are not broadly representative of the residential facilities in Ireland. As pointed out previously (Section 4.2), practically all the residential accommodation in Ireland has been provided by the mental health services and thus, while there may be slight differences between local areas, the method of care and treatment is similar throughout the country. Thus, the recommendations made in Chapter 11 apply to all residential accommodation in Ireland which must take into account the needs of the local area and service users.

One of the prime aims of this study was to investigate the residents' views of their lives and self-reports of quality of life and satisfaction with treatment and care. Practically all residents were happy in their current accommodation. However, if given a choice, a number of residents would rather be at home or in independent accommodation. The vast majority of residents perceived their lives in the residences positively. They perceived that they had control over their lives and could lead their lives as they wanted. Perceptions of their life in the community were also positive. The residents were mostly satisfied with the treatment and care provided in the residences. They also rated their quality of life positively, with the majority of residents 'mostly satisfied' with the way things were. However, as previously mentioned, this must be compared with the findings from the open-ended questions, whereby the perceptions of the residents somewhat differed from the responses to the questionnaire measures. Responses to the open-ended questions showed that residents had hopes and expectations for the future that involved taking more control of their lives and gaining independence from services. It is possible that these anomalies occurred because of a failure on the part of the residents to see

a change in a system that they have become accustomed to, their unwillingness to be 'negative' towards those who have provided them with care and treatment over long periods of time and with whom they had established a close relationship and the lack of alternative options available to them. It is important that service users' hopes and aspirations for the future should be part of the individualised care planning process. In addition, many of the staff had worked in the system for long periods of time and they also may have failed to see the system as one that emphasised recovery as opposed to maintenance. This highlights the need for the training and education for all in community residential facilities in the competences and principles of recovery.

There were significant differences in the clinical and psychosocial functioning of the residents in high, medium and low support residences, with high support residents having lower functioning than those in medium or low. However the clinical significance of these differences is questionable. The mean scores of all groups fell within the mild to moderate range of clinical symptoms and disabilities in psychosocial functioning scores were also in the mild to moderate range. This brings into question the basis upon which residents were assigned to these levels of support. The low level of movement from original placements also suggests that there was a tendency for residents to remain in original placements.

Just over half of the residences had formal assessments of residents, but did not have a full multidisciplinary team to do this assessment, which may have resulted in the inappropriate placement of some residents. While the majority of residences were reported to have a care plans system in use, the residents did not seem to be aware of this. The purposes of care plans are to detail the residents' aims and goals of treatment and rehabilitation. In addition, rehabilitation programmes seemed to be offered on a group basis and not tailored to meet the needs of the individual residents. Nevertheless, the nursing staff within the residences must be commended for their provision of interventions aimed at rehabilitation. This must have been especially difficulty given the lack of training aimed specifically at rehabilitation and the lack of a rehabilitation and recovery mental health team. The two rehabilitation and recovery mental health teams that were in place were under-staffed and did not have the proper skill mix for the team to run efficiently and effectively. The finding that few residents were in employment, either sheltered or mainstream, and the apparent lack of the residents' integration into the community in which they lived suggested that the interventions aimed at rehabilitation to lower levels of support or independent living were not meeting the needs of the residents.

CHAPTER 11
The Way Forward: Recommendations

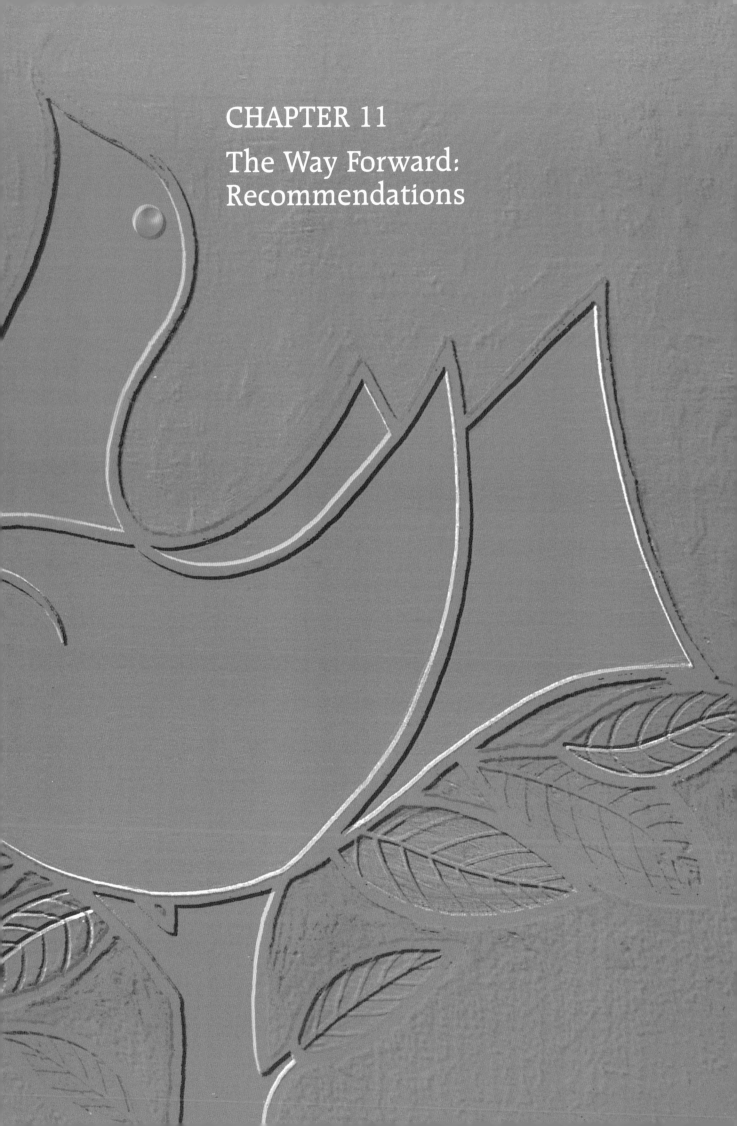

Chapter 11

The way forward: recommendations

This chapter will make specific recommendations regarding the future development of the community residences based on the findings of the study and the information and experience gathered during the fieldwork. The study recommendations take into account the two most relevant recent Irish documents, *A Vision for Change* and *The Report of the Inspector of Mental Health Services 2005* (MHC, 2006c) and evidence-based practice. The authors were mindful of the feasibility of implementing the recommendations within the Irish mental health services and were of the opinion that the recommendations should be addressed in the short to medium term, without delay. It is the authors' intention however, that these recommendations will be evaluated in light of local area needs, requirements and resources and adapted and implemented accordingly.

The recommendations are organised under three main headings: the way forward for rehabilitation and recovery, the way forward for community residences, and future provision of housing for those with mental health problems. In addition, recommendations are made regarding the best way forward for the implementation of these recommendations. Many of the recommendations from the present study are dependent on the implementation of the multidisciplinary rehabilitation and recovery mental health teams advocated in *A Vision for Change,* and these must be implemented as soon as possible.

11.1 THE WAY FORWARD FOR REHABILITATION AND RECOVERY

- As highlighted above, the first step in developing rehabilitation and recovery services is the provision of properly staffed multidisciplinary rehabilitation and recovery mental health teams, which should be put in place as soon as possible.

- All members of the rehabilitation and recovery mental health team should be trained in the competencies and principles of recovery.

- Residents currently in the residences should receive a full multidisciplinary assessment, as should potential residents.

- Staff should, by attitude and practice, orient residents towards raising their expectations of their capabilities to achieve independence.

- Care plans should be developed in consultation with residents, and these should be reviewed on a regular basis. It is imperative that residents are actively encouraged to partake in the care planning process. If necessary, an advocate should be present.

- A key worker system should be in place in all residences and the resident should be made aware of this system.

- The pharmacological treatment of residents should be monitored regularly and residents should be able to make informed choices about their medication.

- Rehabilitative activities should be tailored to meet the needs of the individual, and linked to care plans and should be offered in community facilities whenever possible. The development of these activities should be informed by, and evaluated with reference to, best practice the extent to which they are meeting the needs of the residents.

- Residents who are able should be encouraged to look after their own finances. This means collecting money at the post office, saving money, and having the independence to spend their money as they wish.

- Residents should be encouraged to attend social amenities and events in the community. Those who have difficulty integrating into the community should be provided with specific programmes that address these needs. It is imperative that residents are encouraged to participate in social activities provided by local services and community groups.

- Residents should be encouraged to use and develop support networks from outside the residences. The inclusion and participation of relatives and friends in the day-to -day activities of the residences and in the treatment and care of the resident, may help develop these support systems.

☐ Participation in mainstream employment should be encouraged and the 'place and train' model should be evaluated in the Irish context. For this to be realised, interagency co-operation between mental health services, training agencies and employers needs to be developed.

☐ For those who cannot or do not want to enter mainstream employment, other options for meaningful activities should be provided. These could take the form of voluntary work, pursuit of hobbies, further training or further education.

11.2 THE WAY FORWARD FOR CURRENT RESIDENCES

☐ Community residences should not be used for purposes other than support and rehabilitation. The use of beds for temporary respite, crisis care or emergency transfers in place of acute care is not in the best interests of those who live in the residences. Other provisions should be made for these groups.

☐ All staff working in community residences and those working with this population should be trained in the competencies and principles of recovery.

☐ The rules and regulations of the residences should be re-visited. While some general rules and regulations are required, those regarding the freedom of the residents should be amended to meet individual needs. The residences should provide as homelike an environment as possible.

☐ The aims and functions of the community residences should be standardised so that both staff and residents are aware of their responsibilities to meet these aims and functions. Furthermore the aims and functions of the different levels of

support should be specified and standardised throughout the country and residents informed of these. Currently the residences are providing two main functions – continuing care, and rehabilitation to more independent settings. It is debatable as to whether the alliance of two apparently conflicting functions is the best way to meet the needs of the different residents. The findings of the current study would suggest that the needs of those who wish to move to lower levels of support but need intensive rehabilitation are not being met.

☐ The rate of provision of places, particularly of high support residential places (76 per 100,000), is higher than the recommended 30 places per 100,000 by *A Vision for Change*. The authors acknowledge that a small minority of individuals will continue to need high support care and that some of the current high support residences should be maintained for these purposes. It is also acknowledged that, in some areas, patients still remain in psychiatric hospitals and will need relocation to alternative residences. Residents who have been relocated to community settings from psychiatric hospitals or those who have spent long periods of time in their current accommodation should have the right to remain in these facilities, if they so wish. Newer residents or potential residents should be informed of the temporary nature of their placement and should be encouraged and supported to prepare for more independent living.

☐ As outlined in Chapter 10, the functions of some of the high support residences may change in line with recommendations from *A Vision for Change* (i.e. intensive rehabilitation places, crisis care places). Community residences that will be no longer needed for current purposes can be re-designed to provide for other functions such as intensive rehabilitation, crisis care and high support care. Mental health services should keep this housing stock in mind when addressing the needs of future community requirements, such as mental health centres as recommended in *A Vision for Change*.

☐ The number of places in many individual high support residences is at present above the recommended ten advocated in *A Vision for Change*. The number of places per residence has implications for the privacy of the occupants. All high support residences should reduce the number of places to the recommended level. No residents should have to share a room with more than one person and, if at all possible, single rooms should be provided. If the environment allows, bedrooms should be renovated to include en-suite bathrooms or shower rooms.

☐ The nursing staff resources currently employed in the residences should be evaluated in terms of the need for nursing and non-nursing staff and the current blend of skill mix. Excess nursing staff currently employed in the residences should be re-allocated to community mental health teams.

☐ The health and safety regulations and, in particular, Hazard Analysis and Critical Control Points (HACCP) should be revisited. These currently prevent residents from using kitchen facilities in high support residences, an important aspect of independence.

☐ Evaluation and review procedures to monitor quality should be implemented in all residences. These should take account of the residents' satisfaction and, wherever possible, the relatives' views.

☐ Any outstanding issues in relation to payment of rent should be finalised to avoid any distress to residents, staff and management.

☐ Local authorities have a responsibility to provide nearly 2,000 housing places in medium and low support residences. Intersectoral and interagency collaboration is needed to stimulate local authorities to start providing the 2,000 places identified as needed. The

Departments of Health and Environment, local housing authorities, the HSE and voluntary agencies need to work together to set up innovative, imaginative and pilot partnerships schemes to provide accommodation for those with medium and low support needs.

☐ The possibility of the local housing authorities taking over responsibility for the provision and management of low support residences should be discussed with representatives from relevant stakeholder groups and service users at a national level.

☐ The possibility of voluntary agencies taking a greater role in the provision of medium support residences should be encouraged, with the setting up of pilot partnership projects involving all stakeholders.

☐ Mental health services should contact local housing authorities to determine the possibility of setting up pilot housing projects for groups of three to four individuals. At least two pilot areas in Ireland should be selected and evaluated. The Dublin City Council has already expressed interest in such an initiative.

11.3 FUTURE PROVISION OF HOUSING

☐ Housing for those with mental health difficulties must be provided in mainstream housing in the community. The provision of housing is not the responsibility of the mental health services. As reported in *A Vision for Change* the 'statutory responsibility to provide this housing is not within the remit of the mental health services or the HSE'.

☐ The future provision of housing, in particular medium and low support housing, for those with mental health problems should not be the responsibility of the mental health services. There is a need for statutory and non-statutory bodies to work in collaboration with mental health services to define their roles in relation to the needs and support requirements of this population. Some examples have been provided in the report and these should be evaluated within the Irish context. The authors acknowledge that building effective interagency partnerships will take time. Yet this should begin as soon as possible with those at the highest level of the HSE and governmental bodies providing leadership and direction to those at local level.

□ Interagency working will be most effective when the roles and responsibilities of each agency are clearly defined. In addition, agencies must have mutual trust, respect and understanding of their respective roles and responsibilities.

□ Voluntary agencies, working closely with mental health services and service users, have begun to provide housing and care for vulnerable groups and these existing models should be evaluated and if effective, publicly encouraged and promoted by government.

□ A range of housing alternatives is necessary for those with differing levels of need and support requirements. In contrast to what is currently provided, the level of support should be flexible. Provision of support by 'recovery guides' (as in the STEER project) should be evaluated as a possible model for the provision of low to medium levels of support.

□ All future housing for those with mental health problems should be designed with the principles of recovery in mind. All residents sharing accommodation should have their own en-suite bedroom. All new housing should be life-time adaptable.

11.4 IMPLEMENTATION ACTION PLAN

□ To enable implementation to proceed rapidly, intersectoral action plans are needed at central and local levels.

□ Local groups, one for each catchment area of approximately 300,000 population as recommended in *A Vision for Change*, should have the appropriate representation of housing and mental health interests that will draw up action plans at local level and report to the central group.

□ At central level an intersectoral implementation group should be formed. This group might comprise the following stakeholders - the Department of the Environment, Heritage and Local Government, the Department of Health and Children, the HSE, Mental Health Commission, local housing authorities, local mental health services, local housing associations, and representatives of service-user groups.

The group would:

• Lead on the intersectoral policy changes required to implement the recommendations and develop a central intersectoral action plan accordingly.

• Work through local groups to monitor progress towards implementation.

• Liaise in this endeavour with the implementation and monitoring bodies of *A Vision for Change*.

• These recommendations should be implemented without delay. Many of the recommendations are resource neutral but where resources are required they should be made available.

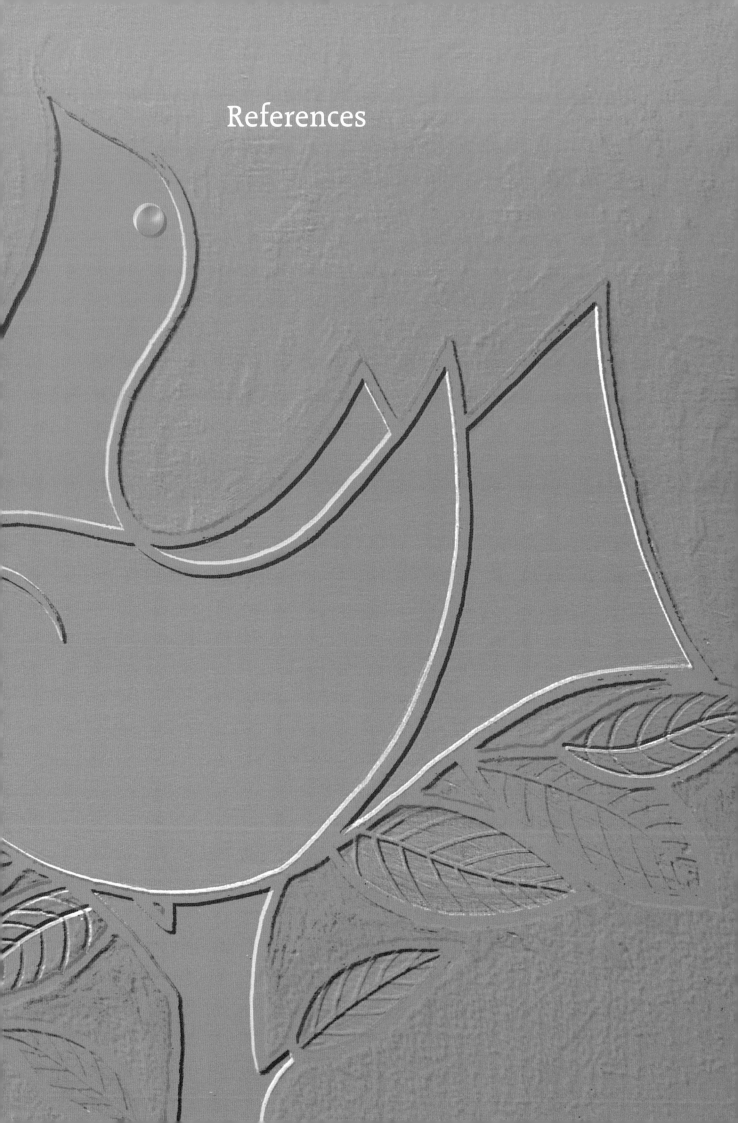

References

References

Anthony WA, Cohen, M & Farkas M (1982) A psychiatric rehabilitation programme, can I recognise one if I see one? *Community Mental Health Journal*, 18: 83–95.

Anthony WA (1993) Recovery from mental illness: the guiding vision of the mental health service system in the 1990's. *Psychosocial Rehabilitation Journal*, 16: 11–23.

Becker T, Thornifcroft G, Leese M, McCrone P, Johnson S, Albert M & Turner D (1997) Social network and service among representative cases of psychosis in South London. *British Journal of Psychiatry*, 171: 15–19

Berzins K M, Petch A & Atkinson JM (2003) Prevalence and experience of harassment of people with mental health problems living in the community. *British Journal of Psychiatry*, 183: 526–533.

Bond GR, Drake RE, Mueser KT & Becker, DR (1997) An update on supported employment for people with severe mental illness. *Psychiatric Services*, 48: 335–346.

Bond GR, Becker DR, Drake RE, Rapp CA, Meisler N, Lehman AF, Bell MD & Blyer CR (2001) Implementing supported employment as an evidence-based practice. *Psychiatric Services,* 52: 313–322.

Bond GR (2004) Supported employment: evidence for an evidence-based practice. *Psychiatric Rehabilitation Journal*, 27(4): 345–359.

British Psychological Society (2000) *Recent advances in understanding mental illness and psychotic experiences.* London: The British Psychological Society.

Brugha TS, Win, JK, Brewin CR, MacCarthy B, Mangan S, Lesage A & Mumford J (1988) The problems of people in long-term psychiatric day care. An introduction to the Camberwell High Contact Survey. *Psychological Medicine*, 18: 443–456.

Brunt D & Hansson L (2004) The quality of life of persons with severe mental illness across housing settings. *Nord J Psychiatry,* 58(4): 293–298.

Byrne P (1997) Psychiatric stigma. *Journal of Research and Social Medicine,* 90: 618 – 621.

Carling PJ (1993) Housing and supports for persons with mental illness: Emerging approaches to research and practice. *Hospital and Community Psychiatry,* 44(5): 439–449.

Commission of the European Communities (2005) *Green Paper: Improving the mental health of the population: Towards a strategy on mental health for the European Union.* Brussels: European Commission and Health & Consumer Protection Directorate General.

Cook JA, Leff SH, Blyler CR, Gold PB, Goldberg RW, Mueser KT, Toprac MG, McFarlane WR, Shafer MS, Blankertz LE, Dedek K, Razzano LA, Grey DD & Burke-Miller J (2005) Results of a multisite randomized trial of supported employment interventions for individuals with severe mental illness. *Archives of General Psychiatry*, 62: 505–512.

Copeland ME (2006) Finding our voice! Ending the silence. Retrieved 26 April 2006 from www.akmhcweb.org/recovery/MaryEllenCopeland/finding_our_voice.htm

Copty M & Whitford D (2005) Mental health in general practice: Assessment of current state and future needs. *Irish Journal of Psychological Medicine,* 22 (3) 83–86.

Corrigan PW & McCracken SG (2005). Place first, then train: an alternative to the medical model of psychiatric rehabilitation. *Social Work*, 50, (1): 31 – 39.

Couture S & Penn D (2003) Interpersonal contact and the stigma of mental illness: a review of the literature. *Journal of Mental Health,* 12 (3) 291–305.

Daly A & Walsh D (2002a) *Irish Psychiatric Hospitals and Units Census 2001.* Dublin: Health Research Board.

Daly A & Walsh D (2002b) *Activities of Irish Psychiatric Services 2001*. Dublin: Health Research Board.

Daly A, Walsh D, Comish J, Kartalova O'Doherty Y, Moran R & O'Reilly A (2005) *Activities of Irish Psychiatric Hospitals and Units 2004*. Dublin: Health Research Board.

Daly A & Walsh D (2006) *Irish psychiatric unit and hospital census.* Dublin: Health Research Board.

de Girolamo G, Picardi A, Micciolo R, Fallon I, Fioritti A (2002) Residential care in Italy. National survey of non-hospital facilities. *British Journal of Psychiatry,* 181: 220–225.

de Girolamo G & Bassi M (2004) Residential facilities as the new scenario of long-term psychiatric care, *Current Opinion in Psychiatry,* 17: 275–281.

de Girolama G, Picardi A, Santone G, Falloon I, Morosini P, Fioritti A & Micciolo R (2005) The severely mentally ill in residential facilities: A national survey in Italy. *Psychological Medicine*, 35: 421– 431.

Department of Health (1966) *Commission on Inquiry on Mental Illness 1966 Report.* Dublin: Stationery Office.

Department of Health and Children (1984) The *Psychiatric Services – Planning for the future. Report of a study group on the development of the psychiatric services.* Dublin: Stationery Office.

Department of Health and Children (1989) *Shaping a Healthier Future – Health Strategy.* Dublin: Stationery Office.

Department of Health (1995) *White Paper: A New Mental Health Act.* Dublin: Stationery Office.

Department of Health and Children (2001) *Report of the Inspectorate of Mental Hospitals, 2000.* Dublin: Stationery Office.

Department of Health and Children (2001) *Quality and Fairness, A health system for you, Health Strategy,* Dublin: Stationery Office.

Department of Health and Children (2003) *Report of the Inspectorate of Mental Hospitals, 2002.* Dublin: Stationery Office.

Department of Health and Children (2004) *Report of the Inspectorate of Mental Hospitals, 2003.* Dublin: Stationery Office.

Department of Health and Children (2006) *A Vision for Change: Report of the expert group on mental health policy*. Dublin: Stationery Office.

Department of Health (2000) *The journey to recovery – The Government's vision for mental health care.* London: HMSO.

Department of the Environment, Heritage and Local Government (2005) *Housing Policy Framework: Building Sustainable Communities.* Dublin: DEHLG.

Donnelly M, McGilloway S, Mays N, Perry S, Knapp M, Kavanagh S, Beecham J, Fenyo A & Astin J (1994)

Opening New Doors: An Evaluation of Community Care for People Discharged from Psychiatric and Mental Handicap Hospitals. London: HMSO.

Donnelly M, McGilloway S, Mays N, Perry S & Lavery C (1997) A three to six year follow-up of former long stay psychiatric patients. *Social Psychiatry and Psychiatric Epidemiology,* 32: 451-458.

Drachman D (1981) A residential continuum for the chronically mentally ill: a Markov probability model. *Eval Health Prof,* 4: 93–104.

Drake RE, Becker DR, Clark RE & Mueser KT (1999) Research on the individual placement and support model of supported employment. *Psychiatry Q.* 70(4): 289 – 301.

Dunne E (2006) *The views of adult users of the public sector mental health services.* Dublin: Mental Health Commission.

Geller JL & Fisher WH (1993) The linear continuum of transitional residences: debunking the myth. *American Journal of Psychiatry,* 150(7): 1070–1076.

Goering P, Durbin J, Foster R, Boyles S, Babiak T & Lancee B (1992) Social networks of residents in supportive housing. *Community Mental Health Journal*, 28: 199–214.

Government of Ireland (1945) *Mental Treatment Act*, *1945.* Dublin: Stationery Office.

Government of Ireland (1995) *White paper on Mental Health*. Dublin: Stationery Office.

Government of Ireland (2001) *Mental Health Act*, *2001*. Dublin: Stationery Office.

Government of Ireland (2002) *Housing (Miscellaneous Provisions) Act*, *2002*. Dublin: Stationery Office.

Harkness J, Newman SJ & Salkever D (2004) The cost-effectiveness of independent housing for the chronically mentally ill: do housing and neighbourhood features matter? *Health Services Research,* 39(5): 1341–1360.

Health Service Executive (2004) *Review of community accommodation within the mental health service in the Northern Area.* Dublin: Health Service Executive.

Heanue K (2006) The need for social housing in peripheral rural areas. *Administration,* 52 (3): 3 – 21.

Hickey T, Moran R & Walsh D (2003) *Psychiatric Day Care – An unused option?* Dublin: Health Research Board.

Hocking B (2003) Reducing mental health stigma and discrimination – everybody's business. *The Medical Journal of Australia*, 178 (9): 47 – 48.

Johnson R (2005) Mental health, housing and community: making the links in policy, research and practice. *Journal of Public Mental Health,* 4(4): 21 – 29.

Jones L (1996) George III and changing views of madness. In Heller T, Reynolds J, Gomm R, Mustan R, Pattison S (eds) *Mental health matters: A reader.* London: MacMillian: Open University.

Jorm AF, Korten AE and Jacomb PA (1997) "Mental health literacy". A survey of the public's ability to recognise mental health disorders and their beliefs about the effectiveness of treatment. *The Medical Journal of Australia*, 166: 182 – 186.

Keogh F, Roche A & Walsh D (1999) *We have no beds…: An enquiry into the availability and use of acute psychiatric beds in the Eastern Health Board Region.* Dublin: Health Research Board.

Liberman RP & Kopelowicz A (2005) Recovery from schizophrenia: a concept in search of research. *Psychiatric Services,* 56 (6): 735 – 742.

Leff J (1997) *Care in the community. Illusion or reality?* Chichester: Wiley.

Leff J & Trieman N (2000) Long-stay patients discharged from psychiatric hospitals – Social and clinical outcomes after five years in the community. The TAPS Project 46. *British Journal of Psychiatry*, 176: 217–223.

Lelliott P, Audini B, Knapp & Chisholm D (1996) The Mental Health Residential Care Study: classification of facilities and description of residents. *Hospital and Community Psychiatry,* 37: 901–907.

Macpherson R & Jerrom B (1999) Review of twenty-four hour nursed care. *Advances in Psychiatric Treatment,* 5: 146–153.

McGee H, O'Hanlon A, Barker M, Hickey A, Garavan R, Conroy R, Layte R, Shelly E, Horgan F, Crawford V, Stout R & O'Neill D (2005) *One island – two systems. A comparison of health status and health and social service use by community-dwelling older people in the Republic of Ireland and Northern Ireland.* Dublin: Institute of Public Health in Ireland, Report No. 5.

McGilloway S, Donnelly M & Mays N (1997) The experience of caring for former long-stay psychiatric patients. *British Journal of Clinical Psychology,* 36: 149-151.

McGilloway S & Donnelly M (1998) Service utilisation by former long-stay psychiatric patients in Northern Ireland. *International Journal of Social Psychiatry,* 44: 12-21.

McGilloway S & Donnelly M (1998) *On the Way to Work: An Evaluation of ACCEPT.* Belfast: N. Ireland European Horizon Project.

McGilloway S & Donnelly M (2000) Work, rehabilitation and mental health. *Journal of Mental Health,* 9: (2), 199-210.

Mental Health Commission (2001) *Recovery competencies for New Zealand mental health workers.* Wellington: Mental Health Commission.

Mental Health Commission (2005a) *Annual Report 2004. Including the Report of the Inspector of Mental Health Services.* Dublin: Mental Health Commission

Mental Health Commission (2005b) *A vision for a recovery model in Irish mental health services.* Dublin: Mental Health Commission.

Mental Health Commission (2005c) *Quality in mental health – your views.* Dublin: Mental Health Commission.

Mental Health Commission (2006a) *Multidisciplinary team working: from theory to practice.* Dublin: Mental Health Commission.

Mental Health Commission (2006b) *Forensic mental health services for adults in Ireland.* Dublin: Mental Health Commission.

Mental Health Commission (2006c) *Annual Report 2005. Including the Report of the Inspector of Mental Health Services.* Dublin: Mental Health Commission.

Mirkin SM & Namerow MJ (1991) Why study treatment outcome. *Hospital and Community Psychiatry,* 42(10): 1007–1013.

Mind (2004) *Not alone? Isolation and mental illness.* [Electronic version]. Retrieved 24 March 2005 from www.mind.org.uk

National Housing Federation and The Mental Health Foundation (1996) *Code of conduct for housing care and support.* London: National Housing Federation and the Mental Health Foundation.

National Institute for Mental Health in England (2004) *From here to equality.* [Electronic version.] Retreived 30 January 2005 from nimhe.csip.org.uk.

O'Driscoll C & Leff J (1993) The TAPS Project .8. Design of the research study on the long stay patients. *British Journal of Psychiatry,* 162: 18–24.

Office for Social Inclusion (2003) *National Action Plan against Poverty and Social Exclusion 2003 – 2005,* Dublin: Office for Social Inclusion.

Office of Deputy Prime Minister (2005) *Supporting people guide to accommodation and support options for people with mental health problems.* London: Office of Deputy Prime Minister.

Picardi A, de Girolamo G, Santone G, Falloon I, Fioritti A, Micciolo R, Morosini P, Zanalda E (2006) The environment and the staff of residential facilities: Data from the Italian 'progress' National Survey. *Community Mental Health Journal*, 42 (3): 263 – 279.

Ralph RO, Lambert D & Kidder KA (2002) *The recovery perspective and evidence based practice for people with serious mental illness: A guideline developed for the Behavioural Health Recovery Management Project, University of Chicago, Centre for Psychiatric Rehabilitation* [Electronic Version]. http://bhrmorg/guidelines/mhguidelines.htm

Rankin J (2005a) *Mental health and social inclusion*. London: Institute for Public Policy Research.

Rankin J (2005b) *Mental health in the mainstream*. London: Institute for Public Policy Research.

Rankin J & Regan S (2004) *Meeting complex needs*. London: Institute for Public Policy Research.

Roberts G & Wolfson P (2004) The rediscovery of recovery: open to all. *Advances in Psychiatric Treatment*, 10: 37–49.

Rog DJ (2004) The evidence on supported housing. *Psychiatric Rehabilitation Journal*, 27(4): 334–344.

Royal College of Psychiatrists (2003) *Rehabilitation and recovery now*. London: Royal College of Psychiatrists.

Santone G, de Girolamo G, Falloon I, Fioritti A, Micciolo R, Picardi A & Zanalda E (2005) The process of care in residential facilities. A national survey in Italy. *Social Psychiatry and Psychiatric Epidemiology*, 40 (7): 540 – 550.

Schizophrenia Ireland (2003) *Towards recovery: principles of good practice in the treatment, care, rehabilitation and recovery of people with a diagnosis of schizophrenia and related mental disorders.* Ireland: Schizophrenia Ireland/Lucia Foundation and Irish Psychiatric Association.

Schizophrenia Ireland (2005) *Media watch report 2004: tackling stigma.* Ireland: Schizophrenia Ireland/Lucia Foundation and Irish Psychiatric Association.

Schizophrenia Ireland (2006) *Talking about choice: developing the dialogue for individual's recovery and partnership.*. Ireland: Schizophrenia Ireland/Lucia Foundation and Irish Psychiatric Association.

Senn V, Kendal R & Trieman N (1997) The TAPS project 38: level of training and its availability to carers within group homes in a London district. *Social Psychiatry and Psychiatric Edidemiology,* 32: 317–322.

Shepherd G, Muijen M, Dean R & Cooney M (1996) Residential care in hospital and in the community. Quality of care and quality of life. *British Journal of Psychiarty,* 168: 448–456.

Shepherd G, Beadsmoore A, Moore C, Hardy P & Muijen M (1997) Relation between bed use, social deprivation, and overall bed availability in acute adult psychiatric units, and alternative residential options: a cross sectional survey, one-day census data and staff interviews. *British Medical Journal,* 262–266.

Shepherd G (1998) System failure? The problems of reductions in long-stay beds in the UK. *Epidemiologia e Psichiatria Sociale,* 7(2): 127–134.

Shepherd G & Murray A (2001) Residential care. In Thornicroft, G & Szmukler, G (eds) *Textbook of Community Psychiatry*. pp. 309–320 Oxford: Oxford University Press.

Shiely F & Kelleher C (2004) *Older people in Ireland: A profile of health status, lifestyle and economic factors from SLAN*. Report No. 82. Dublin: Department of Health and Children.

Social Exclusion Unit (2004a) *Mental health and social exclusion*. London: Office of the Deputy Prime Minister.

Social Exclusion Unit (2004b) *Action on mental health. A guide to promoting social inclusion*. London: Office of the Deputy Prime Minister.

Szmuckler G & Thornicroft G (eds) (2001) *Textbook of Community Psychiatry.* Oxford: Oxford University Press.

Tansella, M (1986) Community psychiatry without psychiatric hospitals – the Italian experience – a review. *Journal of the Royal Society of Medicine,* 79(11): 664–669.

Tansella M & Thornicroft G (2001). The principles underlying community care. In Thornicroft, G & Szmukler, G (eds) *Textbook of Community Psychiatry.* pp. 155 – 165. Oxford: Oxford University Press.

Tempier R, Mercier C, Leouffre P & Caron J (1997) Quality of life and social integration of severely mentally ill patients: a longitudinal study. *Journal of Psychiatry & Neuroscience,* 22 (4), 249 – 255.

Tomasi R, de Girolamo G, Santone G, Picardi A, Micciolo R, Semisa D & Fava S (2005) The prescription of psychotropic drugs in residential facilities: A national survey in Italy. *Acta Psychiatrica Scandinavica,* 113 (3): 212 – 223.

The Sainsbury Centre for Mental Health (2004) *A new model for mental health services in the North West of Ireland.* Ireland: North Western Health Board.

Thornicroft G (2004) Components of a modern mental health service: a pragmatic balance of community and hospital care. Overview of systematic evidence. *British Journal of psychiatry,* 185, 283–290.

Thornicroft G (2005) *Components of a modern mental health service: a pragmatic balance of community and hospital care.* Paper presented at WHO European Ministerial Conference on Mental Health: Facing the Challenges, Building Solutions, Helsinki, 12–15 January 2005.

Thornicroft G & Breakey W (1991) The COSTAR programme: improving social networks of the mentally ill. *British Journal of Psychiatry,* 159: 245–249.

Thornicroft G & Tansella M (1999). *The Mental Health Matrix*: *A Manual to Improve Services.* Cambridge: Cambridge University Press

Thornicroft G & Tansella M (1999) The mental health matrix. A manual to improve services. Cambridge: Cambridge University Press.

Thornicroft G & Tansella M (2003) *What are the arguments for community based health care?* Denmark: WHO Regional Office for Europe's Health Evidence Network (HEN).

Thornicroft G & Tansella M (2004) Components of a modern mental health service: a pragmatic balance of community and hospital care. *The British Journal of Psychiatry,* 185: 283–290.

Thornicroft G, Wykes T, Holloway F *et al.,* (1998) From efficacy to effectiveness in community mental health services. PRISM Psychosis Study 10. *British Journal of Psychiatry,* 173: 423–427.

Trieman N, Smith HE, Kendal R *et al* . (1998) The TAPS project 41: homes for life? Residential stability five years after hospital discharge. *Community Mental Health Journal,* 34: 407–417.

Warner, R (1985) *Recovery from schizophrenia. Psychiatry and political economy.* New York: Routledge and Kegan Paul.

Warner S, Bennett S, Ford R, Thompson K (1997) *Home from home: A guide to good practice in the provision of housing and support for people with mental health problems.* London: The Sainsbury Centre for Mental Health.

Wing JK & Furlong R (1986) A haven for the severely disabled within the context of a comprehensive psychiatric community service. *British Journal of Psychiatry,* 149: 499–457.

Wolff G, Pathare S, Craig T & Leff J (1996) Public education for community care: a new approach. *British Journal of Psychiatry,* 168: 441–447.

World Health Organization (1996) *Psychosocial Rehabilitation: A consensus statement.* Geneva: WHO, Division of Mental Health and Prevention of Substance Abuse.

World Health Organization (2003) *Mental Health in the WHO European Region.* Fact Sheet EURO/03/03. Geneva: World Health Organisation.

World Health Organization (2003) The mental health context [Electronic version]. *Mental health policy and service guidance package*. Retrieved 06 September 2004 from: http://www.who.int/mental_health/resources/en/context.PDF.

World Health Organization (2005) *European Ministerial Conference on Mental Health: Facing the Challenges, Building Solutions.* Helsinki, 12–15 January 2005.

Veiel HOF (1990) The Mannheim Interview on Social Support. Social Psychiatry and Social Epidemiology, 25 (5): 250 – 259.

APPENDIX 1
Facility Questionnaire

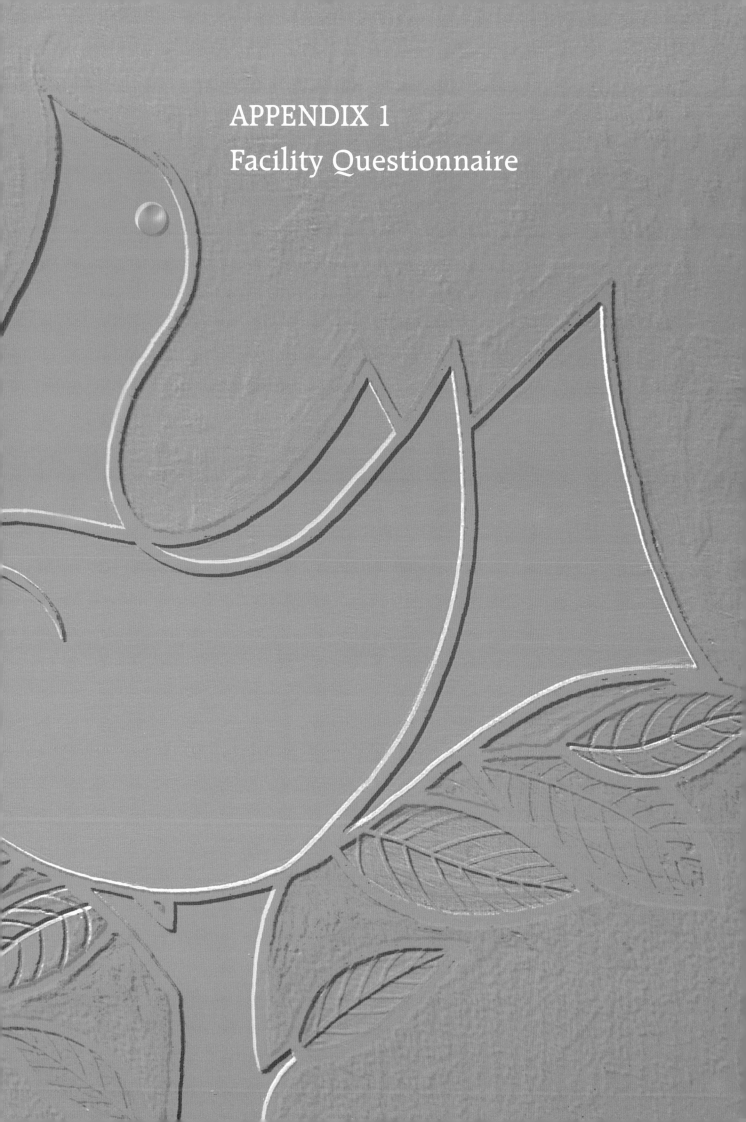

Appendix 1

Facility questionnaire

Name of residence _____ Health Board _____

Date schedule completed ____/____/____   Year residence opened_____

Level of support
High   ( )
Medium   ( )
Low   ( )
Other _____

Completed by: _____ Job title _____ Contact No. _____

Where is the building located
Located in same building along with other residential units   ( )
Situated in a housing estate   ( )
Situated within the grounds of the psychiatric hospital   ( )
Private building on own   ( )
Other (please specify) _____

Description of the location of the building
Urban ( )   Periphery ( )   Rural ( )

Is the building owned by:
Health Board ( )   Voluntary ( )   Private ( )

Building Features

Interior total (sqm) _____
Exterior total (sqm i.e. balcony, garden, etc)   _____
Number of Bedrooms
single _____   double _____   triple _____   others _____
Number of Bathrooms   _____
Number Bathroom for residents use only _____
Number Living Rooms _____
Are there any rooms for staff use only

(e.g. dressing room, bedroom, office, conference room, etc.)	Yes ( )	No ( )
Is there a kitchen?	Yes ( )	No ( )
Is there a designated visiting room (i.e. not TV room)?	Yes ( )	No ( )
Is the building suitable for those with mobility problems?	Yes ( )	No ( )

If no, what are the barriers?

_____

Number of public phones   _____

Is there a smoking room?   Yes ( )   No ( )

If yes, is it   Inside residence ( )   Outside residence ( )

ACCESS TO SERVICES

Time in minutes to reach shopping centre or general shop on foot   _____
Time in minutes to reach shopping centre or general shop by public transport   _____
Time in minutes to reach post office on foot   _____
Time in minutes to reach post office by public transport   _____
Time in minutes to reach pub on foot   _____
Time in minutes to reach primary care centre (GP) on foot   _____
Time in minutes to reach primary care centre (GP) by public transport   _____
Number of residents that have access to own transportation (e.g. car, bike)   _____

Please enter number of individuals with particular form of transport in brackets
Personal car ( ) Bike ( ) Motorcycle ( )
Does the residence have minibus to transport residents?   Yes ( )   No ( )
Is the transport shared with other residence facility?   Yes ( )   No ( )
How long does it take to get to day hospital / centre by minibus / public transport? _____

RULES & REGULATIONS

Do residential staff supervise daytime comings and goings of residents?   Yes ( )   No ( )
Are residents allowed to leave the unit unsupervised?   Yes ( )   No ( )
Do residents have a front door key?   Yes ( )   No ( )
Can residents lock bathroom facilities?   Yes ( )   No ( )
Are visiting hours scheduled?   Yes ( )   No ( )
Are residents required to go to bed at a given time?   Yes ( )   No ( )
Do staff run a check to make sure that residents are in their bed?   Yes ( )   No ( )
Are residents required to be up at a given time?
a) Weekdays   Yes ( )   No ( )
b) Weekend, holiday and bank holiday   Yes ( )   No ( )
When checking out - are residents required to notify staff where they go? Yes ( )   No ( )
Are residents required to check in at a given time?   Yes ( )   No ( )
Can residents stay in their bedrooms during the day?   Yes ( )   No ( )
Can residents lock their bedrooms?   Yes ( )   No ( )
Are residents allowed to smoke in their bedrooms?   Yes ( )   No ( )
Are there any areas where residents can be left on their own?   Yes ( )   No ( )
Can residents choose whom they share their bedrooms with?   Yes ( )   No ( )
Can residents choose to stay in single rooms?   Yes ( )   No ( )
The following items are allowed:
Razor, knife, scissor   Yes ( )   No ( )
Matches, lighters   Yes ( )   No ( )
Medication   Yes ( )   No ( )
Money   Yes ( )   No ( )
Do staff run a check on residents' belongings?   Yes ( )   No ( )
Are residents' belongings listed?   Yes ( )   No ( )
Can residents administer their own finances? Yes( ) Some ( ) No ( )

MEALS

Is the food prepared by the psychiatric hospital?   Yes ( )   No ( )
Who prepares the meals?

	Weekdays	**Weekends**
Residents	( )	( )
Staff	( )	( )
Residents and Staff	( )	( )
Kitchen Staff	( )	( )

Number of residents having their main meals outside residence( )
Do staff have their main meals in residence?   Yes ( )   No ( )
Can residents choose the menu?   Yes ( )   No ( )
Can residents follow a diet?   Yes ( )   No ( )
Do residents purchase/ shop for the food?   Yes ( )   No ( )
Do residents have unrestricted access to the kitchen?   Yes ( )   No ( )

STAFF

Number of daily working hours in residence   ( )
Number of staff for each scheduled shift

Hours	Nurses	Care staff	Household	Others
8am-14pm				
14pm-20pm				
20pm-8am				
Visit daily				
Visit weekly				

Do named core staff, staff this residence?   Yes ( )   No ( )

Do staff rotate at set intervals?   Yes ( )   No ( )
If so, is it   6 Months ( )   Yearly ( )   2 years ( )

Is there an emergency call service in place during night shifts for the residence or group of residences?
                            Yes (doctor-on- call) ( )   Yes (staff-on-call) ( )   No ( )
Does emergency call run for 24 hours including Saturdays?   Yes ( )   No ( )
Does emergency call run for 24 hours on Sundays and public holidays?   Yes ( )   No ( )
Are there volunteers and/or trainees on placement?   Yes ( )   No ( )

ADMISSION PROCEDURES

Is there a formal assessment prior to admission?
            Yes formally structured ( )   Yes but not formally structured ( )   No ( )

How many places are there in the residence?   ( )
Are there any designated
        Respite beds   ( )
        Crisis beds   ( )
        Beds for other uses (please specify) _____

Is the residence ever used to accommodate transfers from
the acute unit due to bed shortages?   Yes ( )   No ( )
If applicable, is there a policy regarding the following admissions?
        Respite beds   Yes ( )   No ( )
        Crisis beds   Yes ( )   No ( )
        Transfers from acute units due to bed shortages   Yes ( )   No ( )

Which, if any, criteria are used as exclusion criteria?

Acute psychotic disorders	Yes ( )	No ( )
Substance abuse (history)	Yes ( )	No ( )
Alcohol abuse	Yes ( )	No ( )
Severe physical disease	Yes ( )	No ( )
Organic brain disorder	Yes ( )	No ( )
Intellectual disability	Yes ( )	No ( )
History of violent behaviours	Yes ( )	No ( )
Former residents of psychiatric hospitals	Yes ( )	No ( )
Former residents of criminal psychiatric hospital	Yes ( )	No ( )

Is there a waiting list?   Yes ( )   No ( )
If yes,
        Number of week   ( )
        Number of applications ( )

Is there a specialised rehabilitation team for the service?   Yes ( )   No ( )
If so, does it have ownership of beds?   Yes ( )   No ( )
If not, who has ownership of beds (please specify)? _____
Who decides on the placement, discharge or transfer of patients?

Specialised rehabilitation team	Yes ( )	No ( )
Individual's care team	Yes ( )	No ( )
Specialised rehabilitation team and patients own care team	Yes ( )	No ( )

Other, please specify _____
If there is a specialised rehabilitation team is it multidisciplinary?   Yes ( )   No ( )
If so, what professionals are included:

Psychiatrist	Yes ( )	No ( )
Mental health nurse	Yes ( )	No ( )
Clinical psychologist	Yes ( )	No ( )
Social worker	Yes ( )	No ( )
Occupational therapist	Yes ( )	No ( )

Other _____
Is there a provisional admitting diagnosis drawn up once a patient has been admitted?
Yes one week to one month ( ) Yes one to three months ( ) Yes less than three months ( ) No ( )

Does each resident have an individual treatment plan with a clear aim?   Yes ( )   No ( )

Does the treatment plan include the following (please tick all appropriate boxes)

The specific medical treatment	Yes ( )	No ( )
The responsibilities of each member of the treatment team	Yes ( )	No ( )
Adequate documentation to justify the diagnosis	Yes ( )	No ( )
The treatment and rehabilitation activities carried out	Yes ( )	No ( )

Are treatment plans reviewed by those responsible
for the care of the resident?   Yes ( )   No ( )

Is there an admission form to be singed by the resident or/and family members containing details on
treatment goals and residential unit process and procedures?   Yes ( )   No ( )

Is there a qualified professional assigned to each resident that
one can refer to throughout treatment?   Yes ( )   No ( )

MEETINGS

Are there planned and regular meetings held by staff within the residence?   Yes ( )   No ( )
If yes how often are they held?
Daily ( ) Weekly ( ) Every quarter ( ) Every month ( ) Very seldom ( ) None planned ( )

Are there meetings between the specialised rehabilitation team and
residential staff?   Yes ( )   No ( )
If so, how often are they held?
Daily ( )   Weekly ( )   Every quarter ( )   Every month ( )   Very seldom ( ) None planned ( )

Are there meetings to discuss treatment and the
resident's response to treatment?   Yes ( )   No ( )

Are there meetings open to residents to discuss the hostel's organisation and
procedures?   Yes ( )   No ( )
If yes, how often are they held?
Daily ( )   Weekly ( )   Every quarter ( )   Every month ( )   Very seldom ( ) None planned ( )

Are there meetings for relatives and families of each resident?   Yes ( )   No ( )
If yes how often are they held?
Daily ( )   Weekly ( )   Every quarter ( )   Every month ( )   Very seldom ( ) None planned ( )

Are there meetings where families of residents can attend together?   Yes ( )   No ( )
If yes how often are they held?
Daily ( )   Weekly ( )   Every quarter ( )   Every month ( )   Very seldom ( ) None planned ( )

EVALUATION PROCESS and PROCEDURES

Is an annual planning report compiled by the residential unit?   Yes ( )   No ( )

**Is there an evaluation plan underlining the hostel's
quality services and control?**   Yes ( )   No ( )

If yes please specify?
Performance indicators monitoring system   Yes ( )   No ( )
Clinical Evaluation of medical conditions
examined by using designated evaluation tools   Yes ( )   No ( )
Surveillance of certain situations or problematic situations   Yes ( )   No ( )
Evaluating residents satisfaction   Yes ( )   No ( )
Evaluating residents' family satisfaction   Yes ( )   No ( )
Integrated Evaluation within programmes
jointly coordinated with other services   Yes ( )   No ( )

Is there a standard clinical and psychosocial evaluation procedure
to assess residents?   Yes ( )   No ( )

If yes, please give details _____

SYSTEM FILES and REGULATION

Are there guidelines or/and regulation in respect of dangerous situation staff may be dealing with, i.e. aggressive behavior; harassment; etc.?	Yes ( )	No ( )
Is there Health and Safety Policy in the workplace?	Yes ( )	No ( )
Is there an electronic fire alarm system in place?	Yes ( )	No ( )
Is there documentation on intervention programmes offered by the hostel available for residents to consult?	Yes ( )	No ( )
Is there a procedure to take into account residents and families feedback?	Yes ( )	No ( )
Is there an information protection act to safeguard confidentiality or/and a freedom of information act for admistration staff when they may have to disclose information to a relative or a representative without prior patient consent?	Yes ( )	No ( )
Is an information pack given to residents on admission (residence rules and regulations of residence, policies and procedures booklet)?	Yes ( )	No ( )
Are residents given information on emergency telephone numbers?	Yes ( )	No ( )
Are the emergency telephone numbers posted?	Yes ( )	No ( )
Are residents given information on rights?	Yes ( )	No ( )
Are residents provided with information on the complaints procedure?	Yes ( )	No ( )
Are residents told the name of the local complaints officer?	Yes ( )	No ( )
Are residents informed of the Mental Health Commission (including role and function in mental health services)?	Yes ( )	No ( )
Are notices concerning rights and complaints displayed on the walls	Yes ( )	No ( )
Are residents asked if they wish to vote, and assisted in voter registration and voting, as necessary	Yes ( )	No ( )
Are residents informed of national health initiatives (e.g. breast screening, smoking cessation)	Yes ( )	No ( )

If so, what information is provided (please specify) _____

Residents Characteristics

Number of residents   ( )
Total men
      18 – 25 years   ( )
      26 - 35 years   ( )
      36 - 45 years   ( )
      46 - 55 years   ( )
      56 - 65 years   ( )
      >65 years   ( )
Total women
      18 – 25 years   ( )
      26 - 35 years   ( )
      36 - 45 years   ( )
      46 - 55 years   ( )
      56 - 65 years   ( )
      >65 years   ( )

Number of residents that have been admitted since…
      < 6 months   ( )
      6-12 months   ( )
      13-36 months   ( )
      ≥ 36 months   ( )

Have any residents been discharged in the last 12 months?	Yes ( )	No ( )

Please specify where residents (number) went after discharge:
Other health unit with higher support ( )
Other health unit with same level support ( )
Other health unit with lower support ( )
Hospice ( )
Family ( )
Home ( )
Other, please specify..

Have any residents been re-admitted after being
discharged during last year?   Yes ( )   No ( )
If yes, how many ( )
How many residents attend a day centre / hospital? ( )
How many residents are in full-time sheltered employment? ( )
How many residents are in full-time supported paid employment? ( )
How many residents are in part-time supported paid employment in the community? ( )

Please complete the number of residents with a primary diagnosis of:

Primary Diagnosis   Number of residents
Organic category
Schizophrenia
Other psychosis
Depressive disorders
Mania
Nuerosis
Personality disorder
Alchol disorders
Drug dependance
Mental handicap

How many residents have a comorbid alcohol disorder _____
How many residents have a comorbid drug dependence _____

Does your service provide the following activities for residents? If so, please indicate the providers of
    the activity and where the activity occurs (*Inside residence refers to activities held in the
    residence. Outside residence refers to those held outside the residence). You can tick more than
    one box if necessary.

Activity	Provider of activity (Please tick)	Location * (please tick)
Vocational training	|__| Nurse |__| Occupational therapist |__| Social groups, volunteers, Other (specify) _____	Inside residence ( ) Outside residence ( )
Sheltered work	|__| Nurse |__| Occupational therapist |__| Social groups, volunteers, Other (specify) _____	Inside residence ( ) Outside residence ( )
Supported work in community	|__| Nurse |__| Occupational therapist |__| Social groups, volunteers, Other (specify) _____	Inside residence ( ) Outside residence ( )

Cognitive behavior therapies	|__| Nurse |__| Occupational therapist |__| Social groups, volunteers, Other (specify) _____	Inside residence ( ) Outside residence ( )
Practical living skills	|__| Nurse |__| Occupational therapist |__| Social groups, volunteers, Other (specify) _____	Inside residence ( ) Outside residence ( )
Social skills	|__| Nurse |__| Occupational therapist |__| Social groups, volunteers, Other (specify) _____	Inside residence ( ) Outside residence ( )
Budgeting skills	|__| Nurse |__| Occupational therapist |__| Social groups, volunteers, Other (specify) _____	Inside residence ( ) Outside residence ( )
Physical activities	|__| Nurse |__| Occupational therapist |__| Social groups, volunteers, Other (specify) _____	Inside residence ( ) Outside residence ( )
Alcohol / addiction counseling	|__| Nurse |__| Occupational therapist |__| Social groups, volunteers, Other (specify) _____	Inside residence ( ) Outside residence ( )
Family education, support, counselling	|__| Nurse |__| Occupational therapist |__| Social groups, volunteers, Other (specify) _____	Inside residence ( ) Outside residence ( )
Leisure activities	|__| Nurse |__| Occupational therapist |__| Social groups, volunteers, Other (specify) _____	Inside residence ( ) Outside residence ( )
Other (please specify, if applicable)	|__| Nurse |__| Occupational therapist |__| Social groups, volunteers, Other (specify) _____	Inside residence ( ) Outside residence ( )
Physiotherapy	|__| Physiotherapist	Inside residence ( ) Outside residence ( )

Activities

Activity	Provision	*Organiser:* **Please tick**
To initiate activities that would involve members of the community	yes |__| no |__|	|__| Nurse |__| Occupational therapist |__| Social groups, volunteers, family Other (please specify) _____

Promote participation in integrated
social activities with the community   no |__|

|__| Occupational therapist
|__| Social groups, volunteers, family
Other (please specify)

_____

Promote participation in events   yes |__|
organized by community groups   no |__|

|__| Nurse
|__| Occupational therapist
|__| Social groups, volunteers, family
Other (please specify)

_____

Facilitate residents going back to   yes |__|
work informally to help improve   no |__|
social integration

|__| Nurse
|__| Occupational therapist
|__| Social groups, volunteers, family
Other (please specify)

_____

Facilitate residents finding work   yes |__|
through employment
agency, regional   no |__|
and local enterprise agencies

|__| Nurse

|__| Occupational therapist
|__| Social groups, volunteers, family
Other (please specify)

_____

Facilitate re-housing   yes |__|
                                      no |__|

|__| Nurse
|__| Occupational therapist
|__| Social groups, volunteers, family
Other (please specify)

_____

Please indicate if the following activities occur

APPENDIX 2
Residents Questionnaire

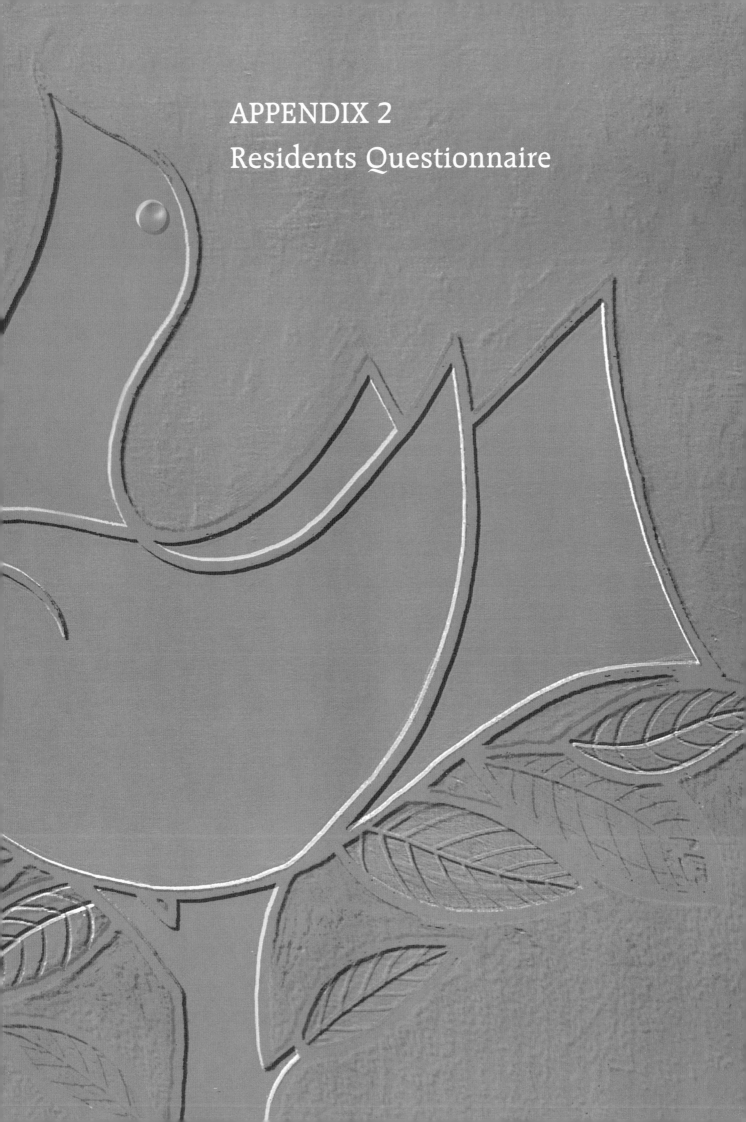

Appendix 2

Residents questionnaire

Site _____ Resident ID no._____ Gender:male ( ) Female ( )

What is your present address? _____

How long have you lived here? _____ What age are you?
_____

| Martial status: | Single | ( ) | Married / cohabiting | ( ) |
| | Separated / Divorced | ( ) | Widowed | ( ) |

Education:	Some primary	( )	Completed primary	( )
	Some secondary	( )	Completed secondary	( )
	Some post secondary	( )	Certificate / Diploma	( )
	One or more university degrees ( )			
	Other _____			

Current employment status:

	Employed full-time	( )	Employed part-time	( )
	Unemployed	( )	Homemaker	( )
	Study /	( )	Retired	( )
	Sheltered employment	( )	Training	( )
	Other _____			

Occupation (if unemployed or retired, what was previous occupation); _____

Do you wish to stay in your current accommodation?   Yes ___ No ___

If you had a choice, where would you like to live? _____

Do you attend any of the following activities in the community?
Social clubs	Yes ___	No ___
Bingo	Yes ___	No ___
Community centres	Yes ___	No ___
Pubs / clubs / restaurants	Yes ___	No ___
Leisure centres	Yes ___	No ___
Library	Yes ___	No ___
Cinema	Yes ___	No ___
Religious worship	Yes ___	No ___

Other, please specify [   ]

Do you know how much money you receive per week?   Yes ___ No ___
Do you receive help with your finances?   Yes ___ No ___
Do you vote?   Yes ___ No ___
Do you visit the GP by yourself?   Yes ___ No ___
Do you go out on your own?   Yes ___ No ___

Have you ever experienced harassment
in the community (verbal abuse, physical abuse)   Yes ___ No ___

If so, could you describe (type of harassment, who committed it, why it occurred, to whom was it reported, how did it make you feel, did it stop you from using community facilities)

If yes, is the harassment continuing?
Yes   ____
No   ____
Occasionally ____

Did you experience any of the following feelings?
Adverse effect on mental health   Yes ____   No ___
Anger and annoyance   Yes ____   No ___
Fear   Yes ___   No ___

YOUR TREATMENT AND CARE

Below are some statements about how you are getting on with psychiatrist and key worker and if you have all the information you need about your treatment and care. From these questions we will be able to gain an idea of how satisfied residents are with the care they receive. Your comments on this questionnaire and all others will be treated in the utmost confidence and will not be shown to any of the doctors or nurses. I will be the only one to see your responses. I will read out the statements to you and please respond to the questions by answering yes, not sure or no. (tick appropriate box and repeat answer options to participant when necessary)

	Yes	Not	Not sure
Your care plan			
I know what my care plan is	☐	☐	☐
I was involved in drawing up my care plan	☐	☐	☐
My care plan has been explained to me	☐	☐	☐
I know what my medication is for	☐	☐	☐
I know about the possible side effects of my medication	☐	☐	☐
I know when my care plan is going to be reviewed	☐	☐	☐
The help you receive from your key worker			
The term 'key worker' has been explained to me	☐	☐	☐
I know the name of my key worker	☐	☐	☐
My key worker has explained to me their view of my problems	☐	☐	☐
My key worker is helping me to cope with my mental health problems	☐	☐	☐
If I have a problem I can easily contact my key worker	☐	☐	☐
My key worker helps me with practical problems	☐	☐	☐
I can easily talk about my personal problems with my key worker	☐	☐	☐
My key worker lets my GP know how I am getting on	☐	☐	☐
I can always rely on my key worker to show up at arranged times	☐	☐	☐
My key worker helps make sure I keep my appointments with the psychiatrist	☐	☐	☐
My key worker makes sure I am alright if I don't turn up for an appointment	☐	☐	☐
The help you receive from your psychiatrist			
My psychiatrist has explained my problems to me	☐	☐	☐
I can easily talk about my personal problems with my psychiatrist	☐	☐	☐
My psychiatrist is helping me with my mental health problems	☐	☐	☐
My psychiatrist keeps me informed about my progress	☐	☐	☐
My psychiatrist has explained how my problems affect my life	☐	☐	☐

These are more general questions (read out responses and tick appropriate one)

How happy are you with the treatment and care you have received?

Very happy ☐   Quite happy ☐   Not very happy ☐   Not at all happy ☐

How much information have you received on your problems?

None ☐   A little ☐   Would like more ☐   Enough ☐

PERCEPTIONS OF LIFE IN THE RESIDENCE

The following are a list of questions regarding various aspects of life in this house. When answering the question please think of how you feel generally. I will read you a number of options and you tell me how you usually feel (**show flashcard 3**).

How good do you think it is to live here in this house?
1 - Not good at all   **2** - good sometimes   **3** – good most of the time **4** - Great

How good is the atmosphere around the house?
1 - Not good at all   **2** - good sometimes   **3** – good most of the time **4** - Great

How well do the people who live here get on with each other?
1 - Not at all well   **2** - well sometimes   **3** - well most of the time   **4** -Extremely well

How well do the people who live here get on with the staff?
1 - Not at all well   **2** - well sometimes   **3** - well most of the time   **4** -Extremely well

Do you ever feel bored during the weekdays or evenings?
1 - All of the time   **2** - sometimes   **3** - most of the time   **4** - Never

Do you ever feel bored at weekends?
1 - All of the time   **2** - sometimes   **3** - most of the time   **4** - Never

How much say do you have in the day-to-day running of the house?
1 - None   **2** - little   **3** - moderate   **4** - A lot

How happy are you with your involvement in the running of the residence?
1 - Not at all happy   **2** - slightly happy   **3** – happy most of the time   **4** -Very happy

How much input do you have with regard to your treatment?
1 - None at all   **2** - little input   **3** - moderate amount   **4** - A lot of input

How much control do you feel you have to lead your own life as you want?
1 - None at all   **2** - little control   **3** - moderate control   **4** - A lot

How happy are you with your level of independence?
1 - Not at all happy   **2** - slightly happy   **3** – happy most of the time   **4** -Very happy

How happy are you with your involvement in the community?
1 - Not at all happy   **2** - slightly happy   **3** – happy most of the time   **4** -Very happy

Satisfaction for Life Domains Scale - Quality of Life
The following questionnaire is designed to gather information on how satisfied you are with specific aspects of your life. You are to answer these questions using one of these answers (**show flashcard 4**) – mostly not satisfied, mixed feelings – about equally satisfied and not satisfied, mostly satisfied. Are you ready?

How do you feel about:

	Mostly dissatisfied	Mixed – about equally satisfied and dissatisfied	Mostly satisfied
The place you live?			
The area you live in?			
Your food?			
Your clothes?			
Your health?			
People you live with?			
Your friends?			
Your love life?			
Relationship with your family?			
The way you get along with others?			
The way people in your neighbourhood treat you?			
Your activities?			
The way you use your leisure time?			
What you do outside for your leisure?			
Services and facilities in your area?			
Your finances?			
Your drug treatment?			
Your life in general?			

DISABILITY ASSESSMENT SCHEDULE (WHO DAS II)

This interview is about difficulties people have because of health conditions. (**show flashcard 1**). By health conditions I mean diseases or illnesses, other health problems that may be short or long lasting injuries, mental or emotional problems and problems with alcohol or drugs. Keep all your health problems in mind as you answer the questions. When I ask you about difficulties in doing an activity think about Increased effort, discomfort or pain, slowness or changes in the way you do the activity (**point to flashcard 1**). Think over the past 30 days when answering the questions and respond using the following scale (**show flashcard 2**).

In the last 30 days, how much difficulty did you have in:					
Standing for long periods such as 30 minutes?	None	Mild	Moderate	Severe	Extreme / cannot do
Taking care of your household responsibilities?	None	Mild	Moderate	Severe	Extreme / cannot do
Learning a new task, for example, learning how to get to a new place?	None	Mild	Moderate	Severe	Extreme / cannot do
How much of a problem did you have in joining in community activities (for example, festivities, religious or other activities) in the same way as anyone else can?	None	Mild	Moderate	Severe	Extreme / cannot do
How much have you been emotionally affected by your health problems?	None	Mild	Moderate	Severe	Extreme / cannot do
Concentrating on doing something for ten minutes?	None	Mild	Moderate	Severe	Extreme / cannot do
Walking a long distance such as a mile?	None	Mild	Moderate	Severe	Extreme / cannot do
Washing your whole body?	None	Mild	Moderate	Severe	Extreme / cannot do
Getting dressed?	None	Mild	Moderate	Severe	Extreme / cannot do
Dealing with people you do not know?	None	Mild	Moderate	Severe	Extreme / cannot do
Maintaining a friendship?	None	Mild	Moderate	Severe	Extreme / cannot do
Your day to day work / training?	None	Mild	Moderate	Severe	Extreme / cannot do

MANNHEIM INTERVIEW ON SOCIAL SUPPORT

I am going to ask you some questions about family and friends that you have in certain situations.

SECTION A. Everyday Psychological Support:

Whom do you like to do things with?
For example, go for a walk, go for a drink, play sport
With whom do you like to talk about things that interests you, such as everyday events, TV, family and son on?

Nursing/care staff ☐   Other residents ☐

Family/ friends outside hostel ☐

SECTION B. Everyday Instrumental Support:

If you had to asked someone a small favour, for example to lend you something, to help out with small household repairs or do some shopping for you, whom could you turn to?

Nursing/care staff ☐   Other residents ☐

Family/ friends outside hostel ☐

SECTION C. Instrumental Crisis Support:

If you had to make a very important personal decision, for example about moving to another house. With whom could you discuss your decision with?

Nursing/care staff ☐   Other residents ☐

Family/ friends outside hostel ☐

SECTION D. Psychological Crisis Support:

Imagine a very close friend or relative is about to die or has died and you just need to talk about it to someone. Whom could you turn to?

Nursing/care staff ☐   Other residents ☐

Family/ friends outside hostel ☐

Brief Psychiatric Rating Scale

Instructions: This form consists of 24 symptom constructs, each to be rated on a 7-point scale of severity ranging from not present to extremely severe. If a specific symptom is not rated, mark NA (not assessed). Circle the number headed by the term that best describes the patient's present condition. **The time frame for the interview questions is 2 weeks. The time frame for the observational questions is the interview period only.** Say to participant; I am going to ask you some questions to do with symptoms, that we ask everyone. When answering the questions, please think of your experiences over the over the last 2 weeks.

	NA Not assessed	1 Not present	Very mild	2 Mild	3	4 Moderate	Moderately Severe	5	6 7 Extremely Severe
Somatic concer	NA	1	2	3	4	5	6	7	
Anxiety	NA	1	2	3	4	5	6	7	
Depression	NA	1	2	3	4	5	6	7	
Guilt	NA	1	2	3	4	5	6	7	
Hostility	NA	1	2	3	4	5	6	7	
Suspiciousness	NA	1	2	3	4	5	6	7	
Unusual thought content	NA	1	2	3	4	5	6	7	
Grandiosity	NA	1	2	3	4	5	6	7	
Hallucinations	NA	1	2	3	4	5	6	7	
Disorientation	NA	1	2	3	4	5	6	7	
Conceptual disorganization	NA	1	2	3	4	5	6	7	
Excitement	NA	1	2	3	4	5	6	7	
Motor Retardation	NA	1	2	3	4	5	6	7	
Blunted Effect	NA	1	2	3	4	5	6	7	
Tension	NA	1	2	3	4	5	6	7	
Mannerisms & posturing	NA	1	2	3	4	5	6	7	
Uncooperativeness	NA	1	2	3	4	5	6	7	
Emotionally withdrawn	NA	1	2	3	4	5	6	7	
Suicidality	NA	1	2	3	4	5	6	7	
Self-neglect	NA	1	2	3	4	5	6	7	
Bizarre	NA	1	2	3	4	5	6	7	
Elated mood	NA	1	2	3	4	5	6	7	
Motor hyperactivity	NA	1	2	3	4	5	6	7	
Distractibility	NA	1	2	3	4	5	6	7	

Can you tell me a bit about what it is like to live here?

Prompts – What are the best bits about living here? What are the worst bits about living here? What would improve living here?
Focus other prompts on issues raised.
Where do you see yourself living in the future?
What are your hopes for the future?

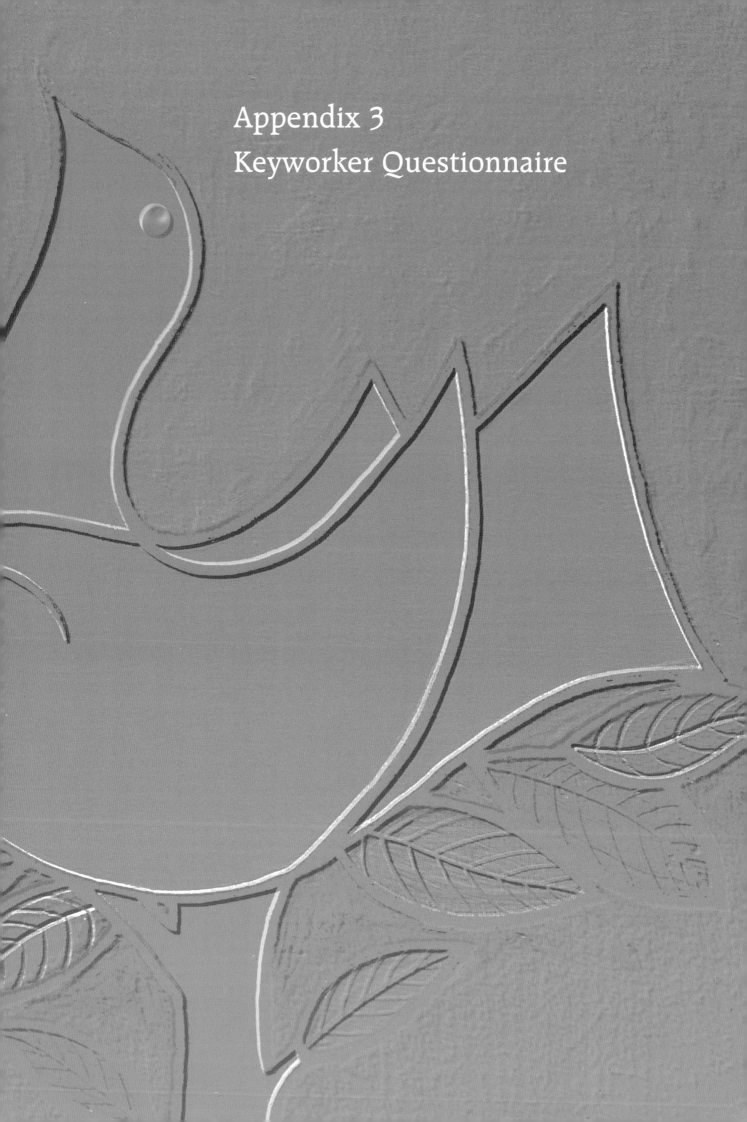

Appendix 3
Keyworker Questionnaire

Appendix 3

Keyworker questionnaire

Site ID _____ Resident ID no. _____   Gender: Male   Female

Former place of residence immediately prior to admission to current residence:

Home ☐   High support facility ☐
Medium support facility ☐   Low support facility ☐
Psychiatric hospital ☐   Central Psychiatric hospital ☐
Acute psychiatric unit ☐   Prison ☐
No fixed dwelling ☐

If answer 'Home' who was the person living with?

Alone ☐   Spouse / partner ☐
Partner and children ☐   Children ☐
Parents ☐   Other relatives ☐
Friends ☐

Income:
Disability pension ☐   *Salary* ☐
Other ☐   *Specify* _____

Psychiatric History:

Date accepted / transferred to residence ____/____/____/

Approximate duration of illness in years _____

Age of first contact with psychiatric services _____

Previous inpatient hospitalisation   yes ☐   no ☐
Inpatient hospitalisation while a resident yes ☐   no ☐

Duration of last inpatient hospitalisation _____

Reason for last inpatient admission:

Recurrence of symptoms ☐   Depression / suicidal ideas ☐
Unable to cope ☐   Behavioural problems ☐
Other ☐   If other, please specify _____

Number of inpatient admissions in the past five years _____

Degree of symptoms in the last five years:
Absence of symptoms   Single episode / complete remission ☐
Numerous episodes / ☐

complete remission   Numerous episodes/ partial remission ☐

Symptoms persistent /
stable   ☐   Symptoms persistent /
                                            progressive deterioration   ☐

Type of symptoms in the last five years:

Psychotic (positive / negative)   ☐   Affective (depressive /
    manic)   ☐
Obsessive / compulsive   ☐   Other _____

Currently receiving pharmacological treatment   yes ☐   no ☐

If currently receiving medication please enter drug trade name, route dosage:

Drug	Route of administration	Dosage (mg)

Please indicate the substances used in the past year, using the following key:

0 = no use
1 = infrequent (1 – 10 times)
2 = occasionally (11 = 20 times)
3 = frequent (21 – 100 times in the year, but not every day)
4 = every day or nearly every day
5 = dependent on substance

	Substance	**Frequency**
Alcohol intake		
Cannabis / marijuana/ hashish		
Stimulants (amphetamines, ecstasy, etc.)		
Opiates (heroin, morphine, etc.)		
Tobacco (number of cigarettes, cigars per day)		

Does this person have an alcohol abuse / misuse problem   Yes ( )   No ( )
Does this person have a drug abuse / dependence problem   Yes ( )   No ( )

System of support in the last year:

Family, friends or other interested in resident and willing to provide support
Family, friends or other interested in resident, but have doubts about ability
to provide support

Potential for providing support, but severe difficulties in putting it into action
Absence of family, friends or other to provide support
Do family / friends visit the resident?   Yes ( )   No ( )
Does the resident go out to visit family / friends?   Yes ( )   No ( )

Participation of the resident in activities in the residence in the last year:

Actively engages, strong motivation
Wants to engage, but motivation is not strong
Passively engages in activities
Shows very little interest or understanding of activities
Actively refuses to participate in activities

Appropriate placement

In your opinion, is the resident appropriately
placed in this residential facility   Yes ( )   No ( )

If no, where do you think the resident would be more appropriately placed:

Independent living: ☐
Independent group home: ☐
Rehabilitation unit: ☐
Low support home: ☐
Medium support home: ☐
High support home: ☐
Nursing home: ☐

If the resident is inappropriately placed, what do you see are the barriers towards appropriate
placement?

Mental state or behaviour precludes discharge / transfer   ☐
Resident refuses transfer   ☐
Relatives refuse transfer   ☐
Facility unavailable   ☐
Facility available, but will not accept   ☐
Facility available, but has waiting list   ☐
Other reason, please specify _____

Where do you see the resident living in six months time?   ☐
In the same residential facility?   ☐
In a higher support facility?   ☐
In a lower support facility?   ☐
In an independent setting?   ☐
With the family?   ☐
Nursing home?   ☐
Other?   ☐

Global Assessment of Functioning is for reporting the clinician's judgment of the individual's
overall level of functioning and carrying out activities of daily living. One score is given in the box
to indicate the individual's current level of functioning. Consider psychological, social, and
occupational functioning on a hypothetical continuum of mental health-illness. Do not include
impairment in functioning due to physical (or environmental) limitations.

Code Note: One score is given to indicate current functioning. Feel free to use intermediate codes (95, 46), e.g., if resident has superior functioning then a score somewhere between 91 and 100 is given.

100 Superior functioning in a wide range of activities, life's problems never seem to get out of hand, is sought out by others because of his or her many positive qualities. No symptoms.

91

90 Absent or minimal symptoms, good functioning in all areas, interested and involved in a wide range of activities, socially effective, generally satisfied with life, no more than everyday

81 problems or concerns (e.g., an occasional argument with family members.)

80 If symptoms are present, they are transient and expectable reactions to psychosocial stressors (e.g., difficulty concentrating after family argument); no more than slight impairment in social,

71 occupational, or school functioning.

70 Some mild symptoms (e.g., depressed mood and mild insomnia) OR some difficulty in social, occupational, or school functioning, BUT generally functioning pretty well and has some

61 meaningful interpersonal relationships.

60 Moderate symptoms (e.g. flat affect and circumstantial speech, occasional panic attacks) OR moderate difficulty in social, occupational, or school functioning

51

50 Serious symptoms (e.g., suicidal ideation, severe obsessional rituals, frequent shoplifting) OR any serious impairment in social, occupational, or school functioning (e.g., few friends, unable to keep a job)

41

40 Some impairment in reality testing or communication (e.g., speech is at times illogical, obscure, or irrelevant) OR major impairment in several areas, such as work or school, family relations, judgment, thinking, or mood (e.g., depressed man avoids friends, neglects family, and is unable to

31 work).

30 Behaviour is considerably influenced by delusions or hallucinations OR serious impairment in communication or judgement (e.g., sometimes incoherent, acts grossly inappropriately, suicidal preoccupation) OR inability to function in almost all areas (e.g., stays in bed all day; no job, home or

21 friends).

20 Some danger of hurting self or others (e.g., suicide attempts without clear expectation of death; frequently violent manic excitement) OR occasionally falls to maintain minimal personal hygiene

11 OR gross impairment in communication (e.g., largely incoherent or mute)

10 Persistent danger of severely hurting self or others (e.g., recurrent violence) OR persistent inability to maintain minimal personal hygiene OR serious suicidal act with clear expectation

1 of death

0 Inadequate information

Insert score here

Physical Health Index

Please rate the disabilities in the following areas and the amount of assistance required, if applicable

Disabilities Key
0 = no disability, 1 = mild disability, 2 = moderate disability, 3 = severe disability

Assistance Key
0 = absence of meaningful pathology / does not need medical attention for this problem, 1 = assume daily therapy without surveillance, 2 = has regular appointments with the GP, 3 = has regular appointments with the hospital specialist, 4 = assumes daily therapy under surveillance, 5 = followed regularly but not daily by nursing staff, 6 = followed daily by nursing staff, 7 = followed daily to medical level.

	Disability				Assistance required							
Cardiovascular	0	1	2	3	0	1	2	3	4	5	6	7
Respiratory	0	1	2	3	0	1	2	3	4	5	6	7
Digestive	0	1	2	3	0	1	2	3	4	5	6	7
Urogential	0	1	2	3	0	1	2	3	4	5	6	7
Motor	0	1	2	3	0	1	2	3	4	5	6	7
Central nervous system	0	1	2	3	0	1	2	3	4	5	6	7
Metabolic endocrine system	0	1	2	3	0	1	2	3	4	5	6	7
Infective (including HIV)	0	1	2	3	0	1	2	3	4	5	6	7

Cardiovascular = to include congenital, ischemic and cardiac valve pathologies, peripheral hypertension and vascular pathologies.

Respiratory = to include conditions like asthma and chronic obstructive pathology.

Digestive = to include gastrointestinal problems including faecal incontinence of any aetiology.

Urogential = to include the urinary incontinence of any aetiology.

Motor = to include motor deficits of any aetiology except that of neurological causes.

Central nervous system = to include particular feelings, epilepsy, the presence of induced tremors or less from substances, and or motor deficits of neurological causes.

Metabolic endocrine system = to include blood diseases, allergic disturbances (reactions), abnormal height / weight relationships, and dermatological problems.

Health of the Nation Outcome Scales (HoNOS)

Please circle ONE number for each symptom as appropriate. Rate 9 if not known. Please base the ratings on the previous two weeks.

1.	Overactive, aggressive, disruptive or agitated behaviour Include such behaviour to any cause (drugs, alcohol, dementia psychosis, depression ect.) Do not include bizarre behaviour rated in scale 6.	0	1	2	3	4
2.	Non-accidental self injury Do not include accidental self-injury due to dementia or severe learning disability.	0	1	2	3	4
3.	Problem drinking or drug taking	0	1	2	3	4
4.	Cognitive problems Include problems of memory, orientation, and understanding associated with any disorder: learning disability, dementia, schizophrenia etc.	0	1	2	3	4
5.	Physical illness or disability problems Include illness or disability from any cause. Include side-effect from medication.	0	1	2	3	4
6.	Problems associated with hallucinations and delusions Include hallucinations, delusions and odd or bizarre behaviour associated with hallucinations or delusions.	0	1	2	3	4
7.	Problems with depressed mood	0	1	2	3	4
8.	Other mental or behavioural problems	0	1	2	3	4
9.	Problems with relationships	0	1	2	3	4
10.	Problems with activities of daily living include problems with basic activities or self-care. Also include complex skills such as budgeting, organisation, shopping, occupation etc.	0	1	2	3	4
11.	Problems with occupation and activities Rate the overall level of problems with quality of day-time environment. Is there help to cope, opportunities for maintainin and improving occupational and recreational skills and activities? Consider factors such as stigma, lack of qualified staff, staffing and equipment of day centres, workshops and social clubs.	0	1	2	3	4

Disability Assessment Schedule (WHO DAS II)

This questionnaire asks about <u>difficulties due to health conditions</u>. Health conditions include disease or illness, other health problems that may be short or long lasting, injuries, mental or emotional problems, and problems with alcohol or drugs.

Think back over the <u>last 30 days</u> and answer these questions thinking about how much difficulty the individual had doing the following activities. Difficulties refer to increased effort, discomfort or pain, slowness or changes in the way they do something. For each question, please circle only <u>one</u> response.

In the last 30 days, how much difficulty did this individual have in:

Standing for long periods such as 30 minutes?	None	Mild	Moderate	Severe	Extreme / cannot do
Taking care of his / her household responsibilities?	None	Mild	Moderate	Severe	Extreme / cannot do
Learning a new task, for example, learning how to get to a new place?	None	Mild	Moderate	Severe	Extreme / cannot do
How much of a problem did he / she have in joining in community activities (for example, festivities, religious or other activities) in the same way as anyone else can?	None	Mild	Moderate	Severe	Extreme / cannot do
How much has he /she been emotionally affected by his / her health problems?	None	Mild	Moderate	Severe	Extreme / cannot do
Concentrating on doing something for ten minutes?	None	Mild	Moderate	Severe	Extreme / cannot do
Walking a long distance such as a mile?	None	Mild	Moderate	Severe	Extreme / cannot do
Washing his / her whole body?	None	Mild	Moderate	Severe	Extreme / cannot do
Getting dressed?	None	Mild	Moderate	Severe	Extreme / cannot do
Dealing with people he / she does not know?	None	Mild	Moderate	Severe	Extreme / cannot do
Maintaining a friendship?	None	Mild	Moderate	Severe	Extreme / cannot do
His / her day to day work / training?	None	Mild	Moderate	Severe	Extreme / cannot do

Is there anything else that you would like to elaborate on in relation to this person? For example, their placement, the treatment and care or clinical or social functioning. Or on factors that promote or impede the individual from achieving their optimal level of functioning? Is there anything else you would like to elaborate on in relation to the roles or functions of the residence?

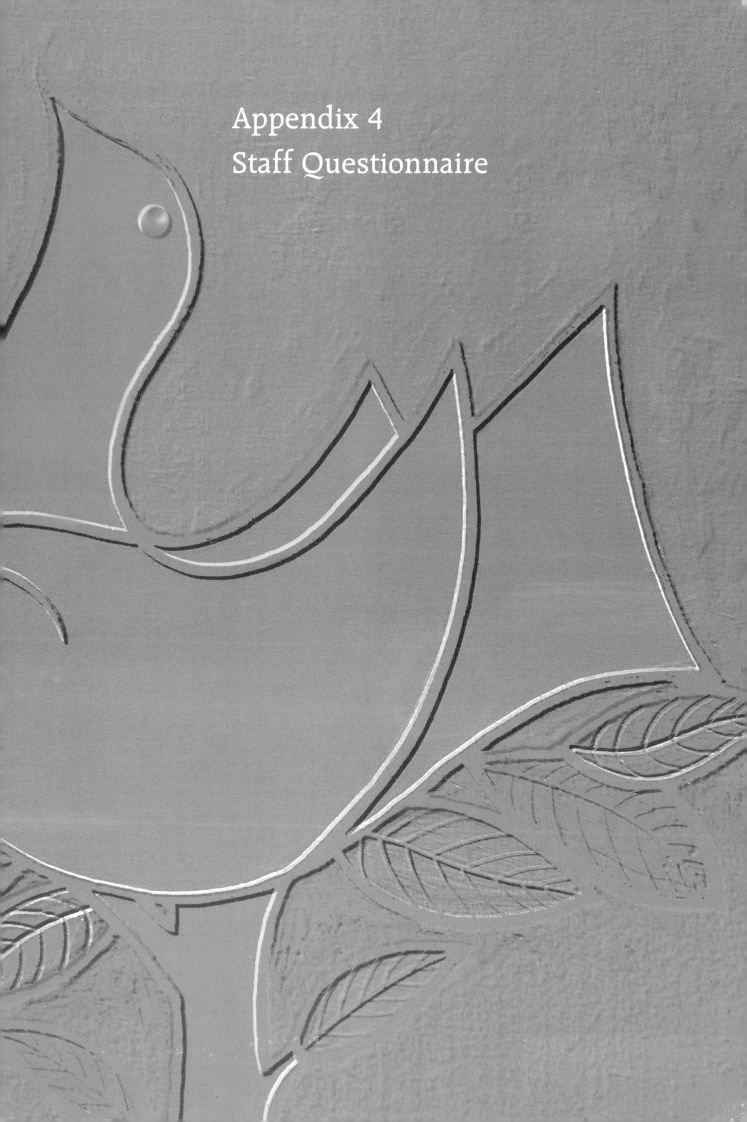

Appendix 4
Staff Questionnaire

Appendix 4

Staff questionnaire

The following staff schedule is designed to gather information on a sample of staff within the residence. One schedule is to be completed for each member of staff selected. The first part of the schedule is designed to gather demographic data. Following this information will be collected on beliefs about aims and functions of the residences and factors that impede or promote independent living for the residents.

STAFF SCHEDULE

Site ID _____   Gender: Male ☐   Female ☐

For how long have you been employed as a mental health professional (in years)?

_____

How long have you been in your current post in this residence?

_____

Which of the following best describes your occupation? (please tick)

Mental Health Nurse   ☐
Care worker   ☐
Nursing assistant   ☐
Care assistant   ☐
Domestic staff   ☐

Other, please describe _____

Which of the following best describes your post in the team?
Permanent contract   ☐
Bank staff   ☐
Agency employed   ☐
Student placement   ☐

Other, please describe _____

Are you employed   Full-time ☐   Part-time ☐   Other

AIMS AND FUNCTIONS OF THE HOSTEL

Please rate the aims and functions of your hostel according to the following key:
1 = no importance; 2 = moderate importance; 3 = great importance; 4 = greatest importance

	1	2	3	4
Service to shorten inpatient treatment	1	2	3	4
Alternative to inpatient care	1	2	3	4
Failure of outpatient care/ day care/ home care	1	2	3	4
Crisis intervention	1	2	3	4
Rehabilitation to independent living / lower level of support	1	2	3	4
Psychosocial rehabilitation and support	1	2	3	4
Home for life	1	2	3	4
Respite care	1	2	3	4

Other (please elaborate)
_____

What are the three main factors that you perceive promote independent behaviour in individuals with mental illness?

_____

What are the three main factors that you perceive impede independent behaviour in individuals with mental illness?